Study Guide

Vickie D. Krenz, PhD
California State University, Fresno

Brief Second Edition

ACCESS TO HEALTH

Rebecca J. Donatelle, Ph.D., CHES
Oregon State University

Lorraine G. Davis, Ph.D., CHES
University of Oregon

Prentice Hall, Englewood Cliffs, New Jersey 07632

Editorial/production supervision: *Robert C. Walters*
Prepress buyer: *Herb Klein*
Manufacturing buyer: *Robert Anderson*
Supplements editor: *Mark Tobey*

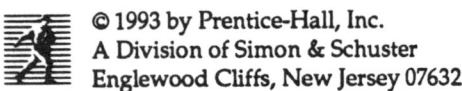
© 1993 by Prentice-Hall, Inc.
A Division of Simon & Schuster
Englewood Cliffs, New Jersey 07632

All rights reserved. No part of this book may be
reproduced, in any form or by any means,
without permission in writing from the publisher.

Printed in the United States of America

10 9 8 7 6 5 4 3

ISBN 0-13-007808-5

Prentice-Hall International (UK) Limited, *London*
Prentice-Hall of Australia Pty. Limited, *Sydney*
Prentice-Hall Canada Inc., *Toronto*
Prentice-Hall Hispanoamericana, S.A. *Mexico*
Prentice-Hall of India Private Limited, *New Delhi*
Prentice-Hall of Japan, Inc., *Tokyo*
Simon & Schuster Asia Pte. Ltd., *Singapore*
Editora Prentice-Hall do Brasil, Ltda., *Rio de Janeiro*

TABLE OF CONTENTS

Chapter 1   Personal Health Promotion: Achieving High Level Wellness   1

Chapter 2   The Foundations of Emotional Well-being 15

Chapter 3   Stress: The Inevitable Reaction 27

Chapter 4   Intimate Relationships and Sexuality 37

Chapter 5   Pregnancy, Childbirth, and Birth Control 51

Chapter 6   Nutrition: Eating for Optimal Health 59

Chapter 7   Managing Your Weight: Consuming and Expending Energy 67

Chapter 8   Aerobic Exercise for Fitness and Health 75

Chapter 9   Muscular Fitness 83

Chapter 10   Addictions and Addictive Behavior 91

Chapter 11   Alcohol and Tobacco 99

Chapter 12   Prescription, Over-the-counter, and Illegal Drugs 107

Chapter 13   Cardiovascular Disease and Cancer: Understanding Your Risks. 115

Chapter 14   Infectious and Noninfectious Diseases 125

Chapter 15   Successful Life Transitions 135

Chapter 16   Environmental Health 145

Appendix: First Aid and Emergency Care 153

Answer Key 159

CHAPTER 1

PERSONAL HEALTH PROMOTION: ACHIEVING HIGH LEVEL WELLNESS

CHAPTER OVERVIEW

Increasingly, people are becoming more concerned with how to achieve health and wellness. Numerous books and magazines give advice on how to improve our health and live longer. However, health is not simply a matter of physical well-being. It also encompasses all aspects of our lives, including the emotional, social, spiritual, and environmental components. At present, evidence suggests that there are benefits to being healthy. The types of behaviors that we practice can significantly contribute to good health. Chapter 1 of your textbook will provoke you to focus upon your personal health and wellness. To help you in your pursuit of personal health the chapter defines health and wellness, points out the benefits of optimal health, examines how behavior is linked to health, and finally presents approaches to changing your health behavior in ways which will enhance the quality of your life.

LEARNING OBJECTIVES

Upon completion of Chapter 1 you should be able to:

1. List the major criticism of the WHO definition of health.
2. List and discuss the four components of the contemporary view of wellness.
3. Explain the synergistic effect of behavior on health.
4. Differentiate between quality and quantity of life.
5. Describe the contribution of lifestyle, environment, and heredity on mortality from the ten leading causes of death.
6. List the essential components you should follow to live a long and healthy life.
7. List and describe the three major categories of factors that influence behavior change decisions.
8. Discuss the relationship of self-efficacy and health locus of control of health behavior change.
9. List the four "musts" in changing your behavior.
10. Describe an overall view of your health from a behavioral or health-status perspective.
11. List and briefly describe the nine steps in positive behavior change.

KEY TERMS

Health
Health Bashing
Health Locus of Control
Health Promotion

Locus of Control
Self-efficacy
Wellness

EXPLORING YOUR ACCESS TO HEALTH

"Wellness Inventory"

The Wellness Inventory is designed to assist you in assessing your level of wellness in the areas of personal habits, feelings and emotions, community, automobile safety, rest and relaxation, and fitness. Place a check by each of the following statements which apply to you.

Personal Habits

1. My appetite is good _____
2. I have an up-to-date immunization record _____
3. I rarely use medications _____
4. I smoke less than one pack of cigarettes per week _____
5. I don't smoke at all (If this statement is true, mark the above statement true as well) _____
6. I drink less than two alcoholic drinks per week _____
7. I don't drink alcohol (If this statement is true, mark the above statement true as well) _____
8. I minimize extra salt intake _____
9. I drink fewer than five soft drinks per week _____
10. I do a monthly self-breast or self-testicle examination _____
11. Women only: I have a yearly breast exam by a physician _____
12. Women only: I have a pap test annually _____
13. I eat fruits and vegetables fresh and uncooked _____
14. I try to eat multiple small meals rather than one or two large meals _____
15. I understand that fiber is important in my diet and know sources of fiber _____
16. I drink enough water to keep my urine light yellow _____
17. I eat a diet that does not require supplements _____
18. My weight is within 15% of my recommended weight _____
19. I minimize refined food in my diet _____
20. I request that others do not smoke around me _____
21. I brush and floss my teeth every day _____

Feelings and Emotions

1. I enjoy my work _____
2. I trust and value my own judgment _____
3. I usually admit my mistakes and learn from them _____
4. Although I value my own opinion, I can appreciate the views of others _____
5. I usually know how I create my feelings _____
6. I know how to change my feelings _____
7. I can recognize and accept my feelings of mad, sad, glad, and frightened _____
8. I know feelings are often transient _____
9. I know how to deal with my feelings _____
10. I can set limits for myself and stick to them _____
11. I can say no without feeling guilty _____

12. I like being complimented for jobs well done _____
13. I think it is okay to cry _____
14. I try to accept constructive criticism without reacting defensively _____
15. I feel enthusiastic about life _____
16. I find it easy to laugh _____
17. I would feel comfortable seeking professional help if unable to deal with my feelings _____
18. I enjoy my family _____
19. I am able to give and receive love _____
20. I can accept the responsibility for my actions _____
21. I set realistic objectives for myself _____
22. I can make and maintain friendships _____

Community

1. I do not waste energy _____
2. I do not pollute the air _____
3. If I see a safety hazard, I will attempt to warn others or correct the problem _____
4. I use nonpolluting detergents _____
5. I would report a crime I observed _____
6. I contribute my time and money to community projects _____
7. I try to get to know my neighbors _____
8. I belong to a group other than a school or work affiliation _____

Automobile Safety

1. I never drink or use drugs while driving _____
2. I never ride with drivers who drink or use drugs while driving _____
3. I wear safety belts 90% or more of the time I am in a vehicle _____
4. I wear a safety belt and shoulder harness 90% or more of the time I am in a vehicle _____
5. I stay within five mph of the speed limit _____
6. I have taken a course in driver education or defensive driving _____
7. I stop on yellow if light is changing _____
8. I use radial tires _____
9. For every ten mph of speed I maintain one car length distance between cars _____

Rest and Relaxation

1. I enjoy my life _____
2. I usually have plenty of energy _____
3. I fall asleep easily _____
4. I can usually go right back to sleep if awakened _____
5. I usually meet my need for sleep _____
6. I rarely bite or pick my nails or fingers _____

7. I do not have money problems
8. I know how to relax my body and mind without using drugs
9. I recognize and meet my sexual needs (Note: There are many methods of meeting sexual needs including art, religion, music, athletics, sexual activity)
10. I have made conscious decisions about my sexual needs based on personal/spiritual values
11. If I were to have sex I would use a contraceptive method
12. I feel my job is ethical

Fitness

1. I know how to measure my pulse
2. My resting pulse is 60 or less
3. I often avoid using escalators and elevators
4. I walk briskly two miles or more a day
5. I bike or swim or exercise vigorously at least one hour per day three or more times per week
6. My daily activities include moderate physical effort (such as rearing young children, gardening, scrubbing floors, or work which involves being on my feet)
7. My daily activities include vigorous physical effort (such as heavy construction work, farming, moving objects by hand, etc.)
8. I run at least one mile twice a week (or equivalent aerobic exercise)
9. I run at least one mile four times a week or equivalent (If this statement is true, mark the item above true as well)
10. I regularly walk or ride a bike for exercise
11. I participate in a strenuous sport at least once a week
12. I participate in a strenuous sport more than once a week (If this statement is true, mark the item above true as well)
13. I do yoga or some type of stretching exercise for 15 to 20 minutes at least twice per week
14. I do yoga or some type of stretching exercise for 15 to 20 minutes at least four times a week (If this statement is true, mark the item above true as well)

Scoring

Count the number of checks in each section and indicate the totals below. To interpret your score and how it may be used to improve your access to health, see the exercises in the section entitled "Assessing Health."

Section	Score
Personal Habits	_____
Feelings and Emotions	_____
Community	_____
Automobile Safety	_____
Rest and Relaxation	_____
Fitness	_____

Source: Adapted with permission of the National Wellness Institute, University of Wisconsin, Stevens Point, WI. Copyright 1984.

"Multidimensional Health Locus of Control Scale"

This inventory is designed to determine the strength of your internal and external beliefs about your health. For each of the statements indicate the number from the following responses which best applies to you.

1. Strongly Disagree
2. Moderately Disagree
3. Slightly Disagree
4. Slightly Agree
5. Moderately Agree
6. Strongly Agree

1. If I get sick, it is my own behavior which determines how soon I get well again. _____
2. No matter what I do, if I am going to get sick, I will get sick. _____
3. Having regular contact with my physician is the best way for me to avoid illness. _____
4. Most things that affect my health happen to me by accident. _____
5. Whenever I don't feel well, I should consult a medically trained professional. _____
6. I am in control of my health. _____
7. My family has a lot to do with my becoming sick or staying healthy. _____
8. When I get sick I am to blame. _____
9. Luck plays a big part in determining how soon I will recover from an illness. _____
10. Health professionals control my health. _____
11. My good health is largely a matter of good fortune. _____
12. The main thing which affects my health is what I myself do. _____
13. If I take care of myself, I can avoid illness. _____

14. When I recover from an illness, it's usually because other people (for example, doctors, nurses, family, friends) have been taking good care of me.   _____
15. No matter what I do, I'm likely to get sick.   _____
16. If it's meant to be, I will stay healthy.   _____
17. If I take the right actions, I can stay healthy.   _____
18. Regarding my health, I can only do what my doctor tells me to do.   _____

Scoring

The Multidimensional Health Locus of Control Scale is comprised of 18 items, with 6 questions in each of the following control dimensions. Indicate your score next to each of the numbers which correspond to statements in the 3 dimensions. Then, add the scores for each dimension. Go to the section entitled "Assessing Health" for the meaning and application of your score.

Internal Health Locus of Control	Chance Health Locus of Control	Powerful Others Health Locus of Control
1) _____	2) _____	3) _____
6) _____	4) _____	5) _____
8) _____	9) _____	7) _____
12) _____	11) _____	10) _____
13) _____	15) _____	14) _____
17) _____	16) _____	18) _____
Total _____	_____	_____

Source: Walston, K.A., Walston, B.S., & DeVellis, R. (1978). Development of the Multidimensional Health Locus of Control Scales. Health Education Mono-graphs, 6, 160-170. Used with permission of the authors.

ASSESSING HEALTH

By now you probably have a pretty good grasp of the idea that your health is determined to the greatest extent by your lifestyle, and that means personal responsibility. The following exercises will help you make the necessary changes in accepting that responsibility and achieving a wellness lifestyle.

1. **Health Behavior Change.** For this exercise you should have completed the learning objectives, the "Wellness Inventory" and/or "Martin's Index of Health Behavior" in your textbook. For Martin's Index, see the scoring and interpretation in your textbook. Also, look at your scores for each section on the Wellness Inventory. Below are listed the average scores from testing thousands of people. Although these will give you standards for comparison, keep in mind that there is much room for improvement beyond the average.

Section of the Wellness Inventory	Average Score
Personal Habits	12.4
Feelings and Emotions	18.5
Community	5.1
Automobile Safety	5.0
Rest and Relaxation	8.9
Fitness	5.5

Now, examine your scores to determine the areas upon which you could improve. Perhaps compare your results from both the Wellness Inventory and Martin's Index. By going to specific items within the inventories you can pinpoint lifestyle behaviors to focus upon in a behavior change plan.

As your textbook points out, many different plans to promote behavior change have been published and no one plan will work for everyone. Your plan might include the steps listed in your textbook. Another possible course of action was suggested by Watson and Tharp (1977) in their book *Self-Directed Behavior: Self-Modification for Personal Adjustment.*

Preliminary Step: From the analysis of your scores on the preceding inventories, make a list of five personal goals for health behavior change. This may include some long-range and some short-term goals as well as some major and minor goals. Perhaps your list would include such things as achieving ideal weight, dietary modification, or engaging in a program of regular exercise. Minor goals might include modifying the predisposing, enabling, and reinforcing factors which contribute to these behaviors.

Step 1: Selecting a Goal. From the list of possible goals you prepared, choose one that appears to be most attractive for your project. Remember, once you have been successful in achieving one goal, you will have the skills to repeat the process for others. Be sure to write your goal as specifically as possible. Then add the following: "I am willing to change my behaviors as necessary to reach the goal I have chosen and will carry out the steps suggested in the following." Then sign your name and have someone witness and sign their name (see the "Behavior Change Contract"). Note that it is likely that your textbook contains chapters or sections which explore topics related to your goals and will provide valuable background information.

Step 2: Specifying the Behaviors You Must Change to Reach Your Goal. These are called the target behaviors. Specify the goal as some "behavior-in-a-situation" that you wish to decrease or wish to increase. You should be able to state your goal as an increase of some other behavior that is incompatible with the undesired one. Specify you goal and behaviors in the following way:

"My goal is to increase/decrease _____ while _____.
                                        (behavior)   (situation)

Initially, it may be helpful to make a list of the behaviors and situations involved in your goal.

Example Goal: Reaching my Ideal Weight

Behavior	Situation
Eating/Snacking	Watching television While socializing While studying When upset or nervous

Step 3: <u>Make Observations about the Target Behaviors</u>. Keeping a diary describing the behaviors, your feelings when they occur, and/or a count of how often you engage in them may be appropriate. You will reveal the events that tend to stimulate or cue these acts and the things that reward them. Keep in mind that the key to self-directed behavior change is self-knowledge. There are several rules for self-observation:

    a. Do the counting when the behavior occurs.
    b. Be accurate in your counting.
    c. Keep your recording system simple.
    d. Keep written records.

A format for record keeping might include graphing your behavior or using the following:

<u>Antecedents</u>: Cues, situations, thoughts, feelings, others with you.

<u>Behavior</u>: Count the frequency of the behavior in each situation and the strength of the urge.

<u>Consequences</u>: What happened? Rewards or punishments?

Step 4: <u>Work Out a Plan for Change</u> which employs basic psychological knowledge. The plan might include trying to alter predisposing factors such as gaining more knowledge, changing your attitude, or modifying enabling factors to make it possible to practice the desired behavior. Your plan may call for replacing an unwanted action with a desirable behavior. You might change the way you react to certain events, or arrange to be rewarded for certain behaviors, or have a reward withheld when you do not stick to your plan. Perhaps you could get a friend or family member to mediate your rewards. A key factor in your plan might be to gradually eliminate a behavior in the presence of certain cues/situations which seem to stimulate it. Whatever your approach, continue to keep written records.

Step 5: <u>Readjust Your Plan</u> as you acquire more knowledge about yourself. As you practice analyzing your behavior and strategies for change, you can make more elaborate and effective plans. Don't forget the importance of record keeping. Records collected in step four can be compared with those throughout your project to easily see the change taking place. This in itself is rewarding.

"Behavior Change Contract"

Name:_____

I agree to

_____

_____

under the following circumstances:_____

(specify where, when, how much.)

_____.

Environmental Planning

In order to help keep me doing this, I am going to: (1) arrange my physical and social environment by _____

_____,

and (2) control my internal environment (thoughts, images, etc.) by _____

_____.

Reinforcements

Reinforcements provided by me daily or weekly:_____

_____.

Special social support provided by "significant helper":_____

_____.

My "significant helper's" name is. (signature)_____.

My signature:_____

This contract should include:

* Baseline observation (one week)
* Well-defined goal
* Simple method of charting progress (diary, counts, charts)
* Reinforcements ... immediate and long-term
* Evaluation method summary of experiences, success, and/or new learnings about yourself.

Source: Adapted from a behavioral contract by Dr. Jerry Braza, University of Utah, Salt Lake City, Utah. Used with permission of the author.

2. **Health Locus of Control.** The concept of health locus of control was derived from the work done by I. B. Rotter in determining that some people have a tendency to be internal or external in their locus of control. That is, some people tend to believe that the outcomes in their lives are most controlled by what they themselves do, while others believe that external forces such as fate or chance have the most influence.

    This concept has been adapted to describe locus of control in terms of health outcomes in people's lives. The "Multidimensional Health Locus of Control Scale" is divided into one measure of internal health locus of control (IHLC) and two measures of external: "chance health" locus of control (CHLC) whether a person would tend to believe that chance/fate (CHLC) or powerful others (PHLC), such as health workers or family members, have the greatest control over his or her health.

    Examine your scores in each dimension of the Multidimensional Health Locus of Control Scale. You will notice that your scores may range from 6 to 36. Since no one is entirely internal or external in the health locus of control, you may have scored moderately high in more than one dimension. The highest score or scores suggests the tendency of your locus of control beliefs. Research to date indicates that individuals with an internal health locus of control may be more likely to behave in ways which facilitate physical well-being. As you textbook suggests, if you believe that you are capable of changing health behavior (self-efficacy) and that your personal actions will positively affect you health (IHLC), succeeding in the behavior change attempt is much more likely.

REVIEW TEST

Short Answer

1. List the major components of health.

2. List at least five benefits of being healthy.

3. Discuss the major factors that influence a person's health status.

4. List three examples of predisposing factors.

5. Differentiate between quality and quantity of life and give at least three examples of each.

6. List the behaviors that will contribute greatly to longevity and quality of life.

7. Discuss the contemporary definition of "health."

8. Describe Health Locus of Control and its relationship to health behavior change.

9. List four "musts" in changing your behavior.

10. List and briefly describe the ten steps in positive behavior change.

Fill-in-the-Blank

1. The process that involves the identification of people who are at risk of diseases and attempts to motivate them to improve their health status is called _____.

2. Lifestyle and individual behaviors are believed to account for over ___% of your health.

3. _____ of life is measured by increases in life expectancy while _____ of life is measured by emotional, psychological, social, environmental, and spiritual health indicators.

4. _____ refers to a person's perception of what forces or factors control his or her health status.

5. List three strategies used by behavior change specialists.

   _____   _____   _____

Multiple Choice

1. According to the contemporary definition of health, which of the following is not true?
   a. Health is an attempt to achieve an optimal level of being.
   b. Health is a static state of physical well-being.
   c. Health is a dynamic process.
   d. Health is a life-long process.

2. The intolerance or negative feelings, words, or actions towards people who fail to meet their own expectations of health is called:
   a. Health promotion
   b. Health bashing
   c. Readiness
   d. Attributions

3. Activities, behaviors, and attitudes that improve the quality of life and expand on that potential is referred to as:
   a. Health
   b. Health promotion
   c. Wellness
   d. Life expectancy

4. The leading cause of death for adults (25-64 years of age) in the United States is:
   a. Cancer
   b. Accidents
   c. Stroke
   d. Cardiovascular disease

5. Which of the following is <u>not</u> a product of good health?
   a. Improved length and quality of life
   b. Improved ability to cope with the stresses of life
   c. Reduced level of creativity
   d. Reduced health-care costs

6. The risks of heart disease can be decreased by all of the following, except:
   a. Not smoking
   b. Increased sodium intake
   c. Regular exercise
   d. A diet low in saturated fat and cholesterol

7. The essential components of a long and healthy life include:
   a. Eating a nutritious breakfast
   b. Sleeping 7 to 8 hours
   c. Limiting alcohol intake
   d. All of the above

8. People are more likely to change a given behavior if:
   a. They believe that they may be susceptible to a given disease or health risk
   b. They believe that the consequences of their actions could be severe if they do not change
   c. They believe that they will benefit from changing their behavior
   d. All of the above

9. The factors that make our health decisions more convenient or more difficult are called:
   a. Predisposing factors
   b. Enabling factors
   c. Readiness factors
   d. Reinforcing factors

10. A person's perceptions of forces or factors that control his or her destiny is:
    a. Locus of control
    b. Attributions
    c. Expectations
    d. Self-efficacy

CHAPTER 2

THE FOUNDATIONS OF EMOTIONAL WELL-BEING

CHAPTER OVERVIEW

In today's rapidly changing society, many demands are made upon us to adapt. At times, our emotional well-being is pushed to its limits and we wonder if we may be "going crazy." Well-being is a complex interaction between the multiple components of health. Our mental and emotional health are not only important in themselves, but also are vital considerations for their impact on our total well-being. If we are to be physically healthy, we must also be mentally and emotionally healthy. Virtually all aspects of healthy and successful relationships are dependent upon one key factor, communication. Chapter 2 explores the foundations of mental health and the theories which underpin explanations of personality. The importance of effective communication in developing a positive perspective of self and positive relationships with others is explored. Finally, the various responses to emotional challenges are explained along with descriptions of coping strategies which are both maladaptive, and more appropriately, adaptive.

LEARNING OBJECTIVES

Upon completion of Chapter 2 you should be able to:

1. Define "normal" behavior.
2. Give a definition of the "emotionally healthy person" based collectively on the views of M. Scott Peck and David Heath.
3. List the eight common characteristics of emotionally healthy people recognized by psychologist Deane Shapiro.
4. Identify the factors which influence the development of the personality.
5. Contrast the views of human personality/mental development held by Freud, Erikson, Skinner, Maslow, and Rogers.
6. List and describe the four components of the healthy personality.
7. Discuss the dynamic nature of the personality in terms of life span and maturity.
8. Describe the structure and function of the endocrine system.
9. Define self-esteem and discuss its relationship to emotional well-being.
10. Identify the "roots" of self-esteem and briefly discuss ways of enhancing feelings of personal worth.
11. Contrast intuitive, creative, and practical problem solving.
12. List and briefly describe the steps in educated decision making.
13. Discuss the importance of communication in close relationships.
14. Explain what is meant by "defense mechanism" and give examples of each of those in Table 2.2 of your textbook.
15. Discuss the use of drugs, alcohol, and compulsive behaviors in defending against or deadening unpleasant feelings.

16. Discuss the problem of suicide in terms of incidence, symptoms, and appropriate responses to a potentially suicidal friend or acquaintance.
17. Describe posttraumatic shock syndrome.
18. Describe the three theories which may account for why two-thirds of all depressives are women.
19. Describe the symptoms of depression and differentiate between exogenous and endogenous depression.
20. List and describe the contemporary approaches to treating depression.
21. Describe manic-depressive mood disorder, its likely cause, and current therapy.
22. Describe Seasonal Affective Disorder and its current therapies.
23. Describe schizophrenia, its symptoms, and treatments.
24. List and briefly describe the various types of mental health professionals and therapeutic approaches which are available today.
25. Briefly discuss what we can typically expect when we begin therapy.

KEY TERMS

Anxiety Disorders
Behavioral Psychology
Behavioral Therapy
Cognitive Therapy
Conditioning
Counselor
Creative Problem Solving
Defense Mechanisms
Developmental Psychology
Developmental Tasks
Ego
Emotionality
Endogenous Depression
Exogenous Depression
Family Therapy
Humanistic Psychology
Id
Impulsiveness
Intuitive Problem Solving
Level of Activity

Lithium
Obsessive-compulsive Disorder
Panic Attack
Personality
Phobia
Posttraumatic Stress Disorder
Practical Problem Solving
Psychiatrist
Psychoanalyst
Psychodynamic Therapy
Psychologist
Psychology
Schizophrenia
Seasonal Affective Disorder
Self-Esteem
Sociability
Social Worker
Superego
Therapy

EXPLORING YOUR ACCESS TO HEALTH

"Self-Actualization Inventory"

This inventory is designed to make you aware of the characteristics of self-actualization. Also, to help you find out whether you are a self-actualizing person, that is, a person who is fulfilling his or her potentials, including esthetic, creative, and spiritual capacities. Circle the number in the column on the right side that you feel honestly describes how you feel or behave.

Characteristics	Very Often	Often	Sometimes	Never
1. Judge other accurately	5	3	1	0
2. Detect falseness in others	5	3	1	0
3. Tolerate uncertainty	5	3	1	0
4. Accept your good and bad aspects	5	3	1	0
5. Accept others even though you disagree with them	5	3	1	0
6. Get creative ideas	5	3	1	0
7. Enjoy doing unplanned and unrehearsed things	15	10	4	0
8. Involved with problems of others	10	7	3	0
9. Able to be alone	10	7	3	0
10. Able to be honest with strangers	5	3	1	0
11. Resist local customs and traditions	5	3	1	0
12. Have your friends support you before making decisions	5	3	1	0
13. Able to make decisions	5	3	1	0
14. Get a lot of enjoyment from playing or socializing with others	5	3	1	0
15. Appreciate seeing a play or concert	5	3	1	0
16. Feel inspired after hearing or seeing outstanding artists/persons perform	5	3	1	0
17. Have empathy for another person	5	3	1	0
18. Help others to grow and become better persons	5	3	1	0
19. Have deep and meaningful relationships with a few friends	5	3	1	0
20. Feel that a person should be hired on ability and competency	5	3	1	0
21. Do work that you enjoy	10	7	3	0
22. Feel that your work is important	5	3	1	0
23. Laugh at yourself	10	7	3	0
24. Look forward to new experiences	10	7	3	0
25. Enjoy peak and unusual experiences	15	12	4	0
26. Believe that honesty is the best policy	5	3	1	0
27. Believe that one should always tell the truth	5	3	1	0
28. Have dedication to life or social purpose	10	7	3	0

Total _____

Scoring

Add the numbers you circled and enter your total score. Go to the section entitled "Assessing Health" to learn more about the meaning and application of your score.

Source: Socochan, W.D. (1976). *Personal Health Appraisal*, New York: Wiley & Sons, Inc. 37-40. Reprinted with permission of the author.

"Beck Depression Inventory"

Have you every wondered if you were depressed or if a friend was suffering from depression? The Beck Depression Inventory is a reliable tool for measuring mood and accurately rating the severity of depression. Although you may not feel depressed at this time, taking the inventory will familiarize you with the areas it assesses, or it may be useful at some time in the future.

Read the statements under each category. Circle the score for each statement that describes the way you feel today. If two or more statements in a category describe the way you feel, circle the one with the highest score. Carefully read all the statements in a category before answering.

Response

1. Sadness:
   I do not feel sad.   0
   I feel sad.   1
   I am sad all the time and I can't snap out of it.   2
   I am so sad or unhappy that I can't stand it.   3

2. Pessimism:
   I am not particularly discouraged about the future.   0
   I feel discouraged about the future.   1
   I have nothing to look forward to.   2
   I feel that the future is hopeless and that things cannot improve.   3

3. Sense of failure:
   I do not feel like a failure.   0
   I feel I have failed more than the average person.   1
   As I look back on my life, all I can see is a lot of failures.   2
   I feel I am a complete failure as a person.   3

4. Dissatisfaction:
   I get as much satisfaction out of things as I used to.   0
   I don't enjoy things the way I used to.   1
   I don't get real satisfaction out of anything anymore.   2
   I am dissatisfied or bored with everything.   3

5. Guilt:
   I don't feel particularly guilty. 0
   I feel guilty a good part of the time. 1
   I feel quite guilty most of the time. 2
   I feel guilty all of the time. 3

6. Expectation of punishment:
   I don't feel I am being punished. 0
   I feel I may be punished. 1
   I expect to be punished. 2
   I feel I am being punished. 3

7. Self-dislike:
   I don't feel disappointed in myself. 0
   I am disappointed in myself. 1
   I am disgusted with myself. 2
   I hate myself. 3

8. Self-accusations:
   I don't feel I am any worse than anybody else. 0
   I am critical of myself for my weaknesses or mistakes. 1
   I blame myself all the time for my faults. 2
   I blame myself for everything that happens. 3

9. Suicidal ideas:
   I don't have any thoughts of killing myself. 0
   I have thoughts of killing myself, but I would not carry them out. 1
   I would like to kill myself. 2
   I would kill myself if I had the chance. 3

10. Crying:
    I don't cry any more than usual. 0
    I cry more than I used to. 1
    I cry all the time now. 2
    I used to be able to cry, but now I can't cry even though I want to. 3

11. Irritability:
    I am no more irritated by things than I ever am. 0
    I am slightly more irritated now than usual. 1
    I am quite annoyed or irritated a good deal of the time. 2
    I feel irritated all the time now. 3

12. Social withdrawal:
    I have not lost interest in other people. 0
    I am less interested in other people than I used to be. 1
    I have lost most of my interest in other people. 2
    I have lost all of my interest in other people. 3

13. Indecisiveness:
    I make decisions about as well as I ever could. 0
    I put off making decisions more than I used to. 1
    I have greater difficulty in making decisions than before. 2
    I can't make decisions at all anymore. 3

14. Body image change:
    I don't feel that I look any worse than I used to. 0
    I am worried that I am looking old or unattractive. 1
    I feel that there are permanent changes in my appearance that make me look unattractive. 2
    I believe that I look ugly. 3

15. Work retardation:
    I can work about as well as before. 0
    It takes an extra effort to get started at doing something. 1
    I have to push myself very hard to do anything. 2
    I can't do any work at all. 3

16. Insomnia:
    I can sleep as well as usual. 0
    I don't sleep as well as I used to. 1
    I wake up 1 - 2 hours earlier than usual and find it hard to get back to sleep. 2
    I wake up several hours earlier than I used to and cannot get back to sleep. 3

17. Fatigability:
    I don't get more tired than usual. 0
    I get tired more easily than I used to. 1
    I get tired from doing almost anything. 2
    I am too tired to do anything. 3

18. Anorexia:
    My appetite is no worse than usual. 0
    My appetite is not as good as it used to be. 1
    My appetite is much worse now. 2
    I have no appetite at all anymore. 3

19. Weight loss:
    I haven't lost much weight, if any, lately. 0
    I have lost more than five pounds. 1
    I have lost more than ten pounds. 2
    I have lost more than fifteen pounds. 3

20. Somatic preoccupation:
    I am no more worried about my health than usual. 0
    I am worried about physical problems such as aches and pains, or upset stomach, or constipation. 1
    I am very worried about physical problems and it's hard to think about much else. 2
    I am so worried about my physical problems that I cannot think about anything else. 3

21. Loss of libido:
    I have not noticed any recent change in my interest in sex. 0
    I am less interested in sex than I used to be. 1
    I am much less interested in sex now. 2
    I have lost interest in sex completely. 3

    Total Score _____

Scoring

Add the numbers you have circled under each category and record your total score for the inventory. To interpret the meaning of your score and its application, go to the section entitled "Assessing Health."

Source: Burns, D.D. (1980). *Feeling Good: The New Mood Therapy,* New York: Signet Books. Used with permission of the author.

ASSESSING HEALTH

1. **Self-Actualization.** For this exercise you should have completed Learning Objective 5 and have responded to the "Self-Actualization Inventory." Review your total score on the inventory and find its classification in the appropriate score range below.

Score Range	Current Potential for Self-Actualization
150 - 200	High self-actualization
112 - 149	Moderate self-actualization
80 - 111	Approaching self-actualization
0 - 79	Below average self-actualization

    As your textbook pointed out, those who search and strive to fulfill their basic needs and move toward self-actualization can enrich their lives and experience life satisfaction. Abraham Maslow (1962) in *Toward a Psychology of Being* reported the results of a study which described the commonly held characteristics among healthy, self-actualized individuals. It was these characteristics upon which the Self-Actualization Inventory was based:

    They are able to deal with the world as it is, not as it should be.

    They are able to accept themselves, others, and nature.

    They experience profound interpersonal relationships.

    They have continuing freshness of appreciation for what goes on around them.

They are able to direct themselves independently of the culture and environment.

They trust their own senses and feelings.

They are creative.

They are democratic in their attitudes.

Reactions: After interpreting your self-actualization score, write in the space below what you have learned about yourself and your level of self-actualization. Compare how you responded to the items on the inventory and the characteristics identified by Maslow and consider those you could improve upon to become a more self-actualized person. Perhaps use what you have learned as the basis for a health behavior change project (see Chapter 1).

2. **Dealing with Depression.** Look back at your score on the "Beck Depression Inventory" and compare it with the table below. As you interpret your score, keep in mind that a persistent score of 17 or above indicates that you may need professional treatment.

Score	Range Levels of Depression
1 - 10	These ups and downs are considered normal.
11 - 16	Mild mood disturbance.
17 - 20	Borderline clinical depression.
21 - 30	Moderate depression.
31 - 40	Severe depression.
Over 40	Extreme depression.

Ideally, we want to have a score of five or below. Progressively higher scores can become "task interfering" and keep us from getting maximum enjoyment from life. In trying to improve your score, you may want to use some proven self-help techniques. For example, practice the "Eight Ways to Boost Your Self-Image" found in your textbook. An excellent source of effective principles and methods for improving mood is Burns, D.D. (1980). *Feeling Good: The New Mood Therapy*, New York: Signet Books. According to Burns, it is definitely safe for all depressed individuals to treat themselves using the methods he has outlined. "This is because the crucial decision to try to help yourself is the key that will allow you to feel better." As you work on a program to improve your mood, take the Beck Inventory at regular intervals to monitor your progress.

3. **Seeking Help.** To whom would you turn for help with something that was troubling you? Identify a friend with whom you would confide and trust. Identify a mental health professional in your community or on your college campus who you would go to for assistance with a problem (get recommendations from a friend or perhaps your physician). List the qualities you would seek in a mental health professional. Visit the University

Counseling Center and obtain information about the staff, programs, and services.

4. **Defense Mechanisms.** Review the defense mechanisms listed in your textbook. Describe examples of when you may have used these coping responses.

5. **Looking Further.** Select and abstract a journal article from the library which reports research or discusses some aspect of mental health/illness. Each abstract should include the purpose of the article/study, the research methods used or major concepts presented, the results and/or conclusions arrived at by the author(s), and your own remarks about the implications of the information for your personal mental/emotional health.

REVIEW TEST

Short Answer

1. Write a definition of the "emotionally healthy person."

2. List four of the common characteristics of emotionally healthy people which were identified by psychologist Deane Shapiro.

3. Describe the view of human personality development held by Abraham Maslow.

4. Discuss the relationship between self-esteem and emotional well-being.

5. Describe the importance of effective communication on the development and maintenance of close relationships.

6. List and describe six examples of defense mechanisms.

7. List four symptoms of suicide.

8. Explain the difference between exogenous and endogenous depression.

9. List and describe three contemporary approaches to treating depression.

10. List the various types of mental health professionals and briefly describe their qualifications.

Fill-in-the-Blanks

1. When a behavior conforms to the accepted standards and patterns of a large group of people, it is considered to be _____ behavior.

2. According to David Heath and M. Scott Peck, emotional health is a _____ process.

3. _____ is the study of the mind.

4. The four categories of emotions include: _____, _____, _____, and _____.

5. _____ is an anxiety disorder that afflicts victims of severely stressful situations such as rape, assault, war, and airplane crashes.

Multiple Choice

1. According to D. Shapiro, all of the following are characteristics of emotionally healthy people, except:
   a. Compassion for others
   b. Has a sense of meaning and affirmation of life
   c. Expects others to adapt to their circumstances
   d. Is able to make health-enhancing choices and decisions

2. Which of the following is not a component of Freud's view of human personality?
   a. Id
   b. Superego
   c. Ego
   d. Alterego

3. The need or desire to be with others or to prefer to be alone is known as:
   a. Sociability
   b. Introversion
   c. Emotionality
   d. Excitability

4. Our sense of self-worth or self-confidence is called:
   a. Self-reliance
   b. Self-esteem
   c. Well-being
   d. Personal satisfaction

5. Behaviors or thought processes that are used to suppress problems so that we do not have to deal with them immediately are called:
   a. Defense mechanisms
   b. Delegation
   c. Avoidance
   d. Phobias

6. Creative decision making is based on:
   a. Our experiences and memories
   b. Feelings or hunches
   c. Black-and-white facts
   d. Unusual or unique solutions

7. The defense mechanism which involves a simple imaginary escape from frustrating, boring, or otherwise unpleasant situations is called:
   a. Projection
   b. Daydreaming
   c. Idealization
   d. Rationalization

8. All of the following are basic emotions, except:
   a. Love
   b. Joy
   c. Anger
   d. Fear

9. The most common emotional disorder in the United States is:
   a. Schizophrenia
   b. Anxiety
   c. Depression
   d. Manic-depressive Mood Disorder

10. Depression that has a biochemical origin is known as:
    a. Manic-depressive Mood Disorder
    b. Exogenous depression
    c. Androgenous depression
    d. Endogenous depression

CHAPTER 3

STRESS: THE INEVITABLE REACTION

CHAPTER OVERVIEW

Every day pressures and demands bombard our lives. Sometimes these stresses can have positive and productive effects or they can have negative and detrimental consequences. Regardless of the outcome, we must adapt to the changes that result from these stresses. Many factors contribute to the stress that we experience and our stress responses, including physiological reactions, psychological factors, environmental distressors, and social factors. Chapter 3 explores the dimensions of the stress response, including the physiological and psychological responses that can have either positive or negative consequences on our well-being. As a part of the developmental process, we experience different stresses and challenges. The approach we take to these tasks can lead to growth-producing eustress or failure and loss of self-esteem. Chapter 3 describes the approaches that can help us to effectively manage the stress in our lives, including behavioral strategies, physical activity, and relaxation techniques

LEARNING OBJECTIVES

Upon completion of Chapter 3 you should be able to:

1. List the multiple factors which contribute to stress and stress responses.
2. Define stress, stressor, strain, eustressor, distressor, and homeostasis.
3. Describe the physiological response to stress with special attention to Selye's General Adaptation Syndrome.
4. Describe the purpose of the cognitive stress system in relationship to stress responses.
5. Describe Type A, B, C, and E personalities.
6. Describe psychological hardiness and how it relates to the Type A personality.
7. Discuss how effective communication can be used to reduce stress.
8. Discuss the role of self-efficacy and control in the management of stress.
9. Identify the environmental distressors that contribute to the development of stress related disorders.
10. List the psychosocial distressors that contribute to stress and stress responses.
11. Discuss the relationship of overload and burnout to stress, in particular the progression of stages in the development of burnout.
12. Discuss the stressors and effects of distress encountered during the various stages of the life span.
13. Recognize and assess the distress in your life.
14. Formulate a plan to reduce and manage the daily stress in your life.

KEY TERMS

Adrenocorticotropic Hormone	Homeostasis
Autonomic Nervous System (ANS)	Hypnosis
Background Distressors	Meditation
Biofeedback	Norepinephrine
Burnout	Overload
Cognitive Stress System	Parasympathetic Nervous System
Cortisol	Psychological Hardiness
Distress	Strain
Deep Muscle Relaxation	Stress
Epinephrine	Stressor
Eustress	Sympathetic Nervous System
General Adaptation Syndrome	

EXPLORING YOUR ACCESS TO HEALTH

"Stress Self-Assessment"

It is important to identify how you respond to stressful situations in order to reduce the negative emotional and physiological effects that can result. Answer each of the following questions about a specific stressful situation.

1. Briefly describe a stressful situation that you have encountered.

2. Did you feel any of the following emotions? (Check all that apply.)

   a. Happy   _____ yes _____ no

   b. Depressed or sad   _____ yes _____ no

   c. Anxious   _____ yes _____ no

   d. Like you wanted to run   _____ yes _____ no

   e. Like you wanted to strike out at something _____ yes _____ no

   f. Angry   _____ yes _____ no

   g. Other   _____ yes _____ no
      Describe:

3. Did you feel any of the following physiological symptoms?

   a. Headache   _____ yes _____ no

b. Stomach upset (including cramps, nausea, sharp pains, constipation, diarrhea) _____ yes _____ no

c. Fatigue _____ yes _____ no

d. Insomnia (including an inability to fall asleep or awakening in the middle of the night and unable to get back to sleep) _____ yes _____ no

e. Increased heart beats, hypertension, or angina (chest pains from heart trouble) _____ yes _____ no

f. Tightness in your chest or difficulty breathing _____ yes _____ no

g. Muscle tension (including in your back, arms, legs, shoulders, or neck) _____ yes _____ no

h. Cold and/or sweatty (especially sweaty hands) _____ yes _____ no

g Other Describe: _____ yes _____ no

ASSESSING HEALTH

1. **Assess Your Distress.** Complete the "Assess Your Distress" inventory in your textbook. Total your points and compare your responses with the scale at the end of the assessment. If your score is in the moderate to high stress range, what stressors can you control to reduce the rate of change you have been subjected to during the last 12 months? Are there any prestress and poststress coping strategies that you could incorporate into your life that would be beneficial? Go to the next exercise in this section (Relaxation Self-Assessment) for further assessment of your stress indicators.

2. **Stress Self-Assessment.** Review the items that you checked yes on the Stress Self-Assessment. Even though you may not consciously feel that you are experiencing a great deal of stress, your physical and/or emotional stress symptoms may indicate otherwise. What prestress coping skills and poststress management techniques (see your textbook) would be beneficial for you? As you learn and practice these new skills, keep a daily log of your progress.

3. **Relaxation Technique.** A variety of approaches of stress management are presented in your textbook. Most of these may be used singularly or in combination as part of a total stress management program. Autogenic Training is another popular approach which has been used effectively to not only combat stress, but to overcome situational anxiety, fears, and phobias when combined with imagery techniques (see 4. Guided Imagery).

You will want to commit the following commands to memory or perhaps record them on a cassette tape. As you practice this technique, sit or lie in a comfortable and quiet place with your eyes closed. Beginning with Phase I (Heaviness), focus your attention on the extremity and repeat each phrase to yourself as you exhale. Once you have mastered the heaviness of your extremities, progress on to the next phase until you have completed each phase.

PHASE I: HEAVINESS

My right arm is comfortably heavy
My left arm is comfortably heavy
Both my arms are comfortably heavy

My right leg is comfortably heavy
My left leg is comfortably heavy
Both my legs are comfortably heavy

PHASE II: WARMTH

My right arm is comfortably warm
My left arm is comfortably warm
Both my arms are comfortably warm

My right leg is comfortably warm
My left leg is comfortably warm
Both my legs are comfortably warm

PHASE III: HEART

My heartbeat is calm and regular
(repeat five times)

PHASE IV: BREATHING

My breathing is calm and relaxed
(repeat five times)

PHASE V: SOLAR PLEXIS*

My solar plexus (body center) is comfortably warm (repeat five times)

PHASE VI: FOREHEAD

My fore head is comfortably cool.
(repeat five times)

*The Solar Plexus is located in the abdominal region of the body trunk between the mid-abdominal muscles and the spinal cord. The term "body center" may be substituted for the phrase "solar plexus."

Note: Once autogenic training has been mastered, it may be coupled with imagery.

4. **Guided Imagery.** Spend several minutes practicing your preferred relaxation routine. Once you are relaxed, incorporate one of the following guided imagery techniques into your practice session:

   a. Record one of the following guided imagery scripts on a cassette tape and play it back as you continue your relaxation session:

   "Imagine a series of scattered streams tumbling down a hillside with a lofty waterfall and some churning rapids. You follow the scattered, agitated energy of the water until it finally empties into a supremely quiet, tranquil pool or lake. The water has reached its level and now has no more need to rush and roar about. You remind yourself, while contemplating the tranquillity of the deep pool, that all of us go along like the water, passing through periods of seething, stormy discontent. And then you see the problems in your life as ripples on the surface of the pool. Get in touch with just how deep the pool is and what a large part of it remains undisturbed by the surface agitation."

Source: S. Didato, *Psycho-techniques* , pp. 45-46.

"Close your eyes and feel your body begin to relax. Each time you exhale, feel your body relax. (Pause.) And as you count backwards from three to one, continue to allow your body to become very com-fortable and very relaxed. (Pause.) Now, imagine yourself lying on the beach in the comfortably warm sand. Allow your body to feel warmed by the sand...Feeling very comfortable and very relaxed. (Pause.). Feel the comfortable warmth in your legs...Allow the warmth to flow up through your legs and into your abdomen...Feel the warmth in your abdomen... Now allow the warmth to flow up into your chest. Feeling very comfortable and very relaxed...Allow your breathing to continue at its own comfortable rate... Now, allow the warmth to flow into your back...Relaxing your back... (Pause)...Feel the muscles in your back continue to relax...And now, feel the warmth flow into your shoulders and into your arms...Allow your shoulders and arms to relax, feeling very comfortable and very relaxed (Pause.) And as you continue to relax, feel the comfortable warmth flow up into your head, relaxing the muscles on the back of your head and scalp to relax...(Pause)...As you continue to relax in the warmth of the sun, imagine that your head is now shaded by an umbrella or tree and your body is comfortably warmed by the sand. Now, take a few minutes to enjoy this comfort- able place. As you continue to relax, take a moment to notice the sounds and smells around you. (Pause.) And when you are ready to return to your normal, awake state, take a deep breath, stretch, and open your eyes."

"Close your eyes and feel your body begin to relax. Each time you exhale, feel your body become more relaxed and comfortable. (Pause.) Imagine that you are walking on a mountain trail. As you walk, notice the sights and sounds around you...(Pause.) As you walk, you come to a clearing that has a lake. As you walk over to the lake, look for a comfortable place to sit or lie down and rest...Take a few moments to rest in this peaceful, comfortable place. (Pause.) Now that you have rested, pick up a few rocks and imagine that these rock are your stresses. Examine these rocks and give them colors that represent your stresses. (Pause.) Now set the rocks back down on the ground and leave them there. As you leave, know that you can return to this comfortable place that is free of the worries and stresses of your everyday life. "

b. As you continue your relaxation routine, imagine yourself performing a particular task. It may be an upcoming class presentation, performing a musical piece, taking a test, or maybe even an athletic skill. Practice the task over and over in you mind, paying close attention to the important details. Also, pay attention to how you feel while you are performing this task. If you notice anything that needs to be changed or could be improved, change it as you practice the task in your mind.

5. **Stress Management Plan.** Review your responses to the previous assessment. Evaluate the prestress coping and poststress management strategies that you routinely employ. Are there other coping and stress management strategies that you could use in the future? As we go through the various changes in our lives, we are faced with different future stresses. Consider the life changes that you will be facing and how you might minimize their stressful effects. Perhaps select stress management as the focus for a health behavior change project (see Chapter 1 of this workbook).

REVIEW TEST

1. List three factors that contribute to stress.

2. Describe the following,

   A. Stress:

   B. Stressor:

   C. Strain:

   D. Eustressor:

   E. Distressor:

F. Homeostasis:

3. Describe the General Adaptation Syndrome and the body's physiological response to stress.

4. Describe Type A, B, C, and E personality factors.

5. Identify three environmental distressors.

6. List four psychosocial distressors.

7. Describe the relationship between overload and burnout.

8. Discuss the stressors and effects of distress during the following stages of the life span:

   A. Infancy:

   B. Childhood:

   C. Adolescence:

   D. Young adults, especially college:

   E. Adulthood:

   F. Older adulthood:

9. Describe three types of daily stress situations.

10. Describe three stress management strategies.

Fill-in-the-Blank

1. _____ is the mental and physical responses our bodies experience in response to any type of change.

2. The autonomic nervous system has two branches known as:

    a) _____

    b) _____

3. The three major traits that contribute to a psychological hardinesss are _____, _____, and _____.

4. A major source of stress among older adults is _____.

5. _____ is a relaxation technique that involves deep breathing and concentrating on an object.

Multiple Choice

1. Any physical, social, or psychological event or condition that triggers a stress reaction is known as:
    a. Stress
    b. Stressor
    c. Strain
    d. Eustress

2. Stress that produces positive opportunities for personal growth are called:
    a. Homeostasis
    b. Strain
    c. Eustress
    d. Distress

3. A balanced physical state in which all of the body's systems function smoothly results in:
    a. Homeostasis
    b. Distress
    c. Eustress
    d. General Adaptation Syndrome

4. The branch of the Autonomic Nervous System that is responsible for stress arousal is:
   a. Central Nervous System
   b. Parasympathetic Nervous System
   c. Sympathetic Nervous System
   d. Endocrine System

5. A hormone secreted by the adrenal glands that is responsible for stimulating the body is:
   a. Epinephrine
   b. Adrenocorticotropic Hormone (ACTH)
   c. Adrenaline
   d. Both a and c

6. The Type A personality is characterized by all of the following except:
   a. Driven by time
   b. Able to relax on vacations
   c. Competitiveness
   d. Aggressiveness

7. Everyday stress caused by noise, air, and chemical pollution, crowding, and urban commuting is called:
   a. Background distressors
   b. Environmental distressors
   c. Psychosocial distressors
   d. Sociological distressors

8. Individuals who feel that their behavior will influence the ultimate outcome of events tend to have a(n):
   a. Self-efficacy
   b. External control
   c. Internal control
   d. Ultimate control

9. Overload occurs when we suffer from:
   a. Excessive time pressure
   b. Excessive responsibility
   c. Lack of support
   d. All of the above

10. A stress management technique that involves self-monitoring our physical responses to stress is:
    a. Meditation
    b. Biofeedback
    c. Hypnosis
    d. Deep-muscle relaxation

CHAPTER 4

INTIMATE RELATIONSHIPS AND SEXUALITY

CHAPTER OVERVIEW

Human beings are social animals, and thus, are continually engaged in developing, maintaining, and ending relationships at various levels of commitment and intimacy. Intimacy involves developing levels of intimate relationships in several dimensions. Making a commitment to another individual is a serious decision that requires a partner to act in a way that perpetuates the well-being of the other person, the self and the relationship. Commitment and intimacy may also lead to sexual relationships. As a part of our sexual development and maturity, we must examine our sexual values and behavior. In light of the vast amount of information available on our sexual development and functioning, there continues to be a great deal of misunderstandings about such sexual concerns as pornography, prostitution, sexual assault, sexual dysfunction, sexual variance, sexual communication, and "good sex." Chapter 4 describes the types of committed relationships and the elements that contribute to a successful committed relationship. While it is the intent of most individuals that their committed relationship is lasting, many couples may be compelled to end their relationship. Chapter 4 also explores the intricate female and male reproductive system, the physiological process of the human sexual response. Further, sexual orientation is explored and how we can develop rewarding sexual relationships. Chapter 4 concludes with a discussion of legal issues that concern sexual behavior.

LEARNING OBJECTIVES

Upon completion of Chapter 4 you should be able to:

1. Describe the characteristics of intimate relationships.
2. Define "emotional availability" and give examples of circumstances which would reduce this state.
3. List barriers to intimacy and explain how basic developmental differences between men and women may account for such obstacles.
4. Define "commitment" and discuss what is necessary to maintain it.
5. Briefly describe the characteristics of the following forms of committed relationships: marriage, cohabitation, common-law.
6. Explain how accountability and self-nurturance are important to maintaining a good relationship.
7. Explain what is meant by "trust," describe its elements, and discuss how to develop and maintain trust in a relationship.
8. Discuss the function of gender roles, power, monogamy, and children in enhancing or ruining a relationship.
9. Describe the warning signs of a declining relationship.
10. Discuss the reasons why couples decide to break up, the consequences of such decisions, and ways to facilitate healing.

11. Differentiate between sexual identity and sexual maturity.
12. Describe the female reproductive anatomy and physiology.
13. Describe the male reproductive anatomy and physiology.
14. Explain the similarities and differences in sexual responses of males and females.
15. Differentiate between homosexuality, bisexuality, and heterosexuality and summarize what may be concluded from research on the cause of sexual preference.
16. Define "masturbation" and differentiate between healthy and unhealthy performance of this sexual act.
17. Explain what is meant by the statement: "Good sex should not be dependent upon chemical substances."
18. Describe the different forms of male and female sexual dysfunction and approaches to overcoming these problems.
19. Describe measures to protect against rape and steps to take following such violations.
20. Describe the two forms of child sexual abuse and approaches to helping abusive parents.
21. Discuss sexual harassment and ways it can be prevented.

KEY TERMS

Accountability	Mons Veneris
Acquaintance Rape	Ovarian Follicle
Anus	Ovaries
Autonomy	Ovulation
Bisexuality	Power
Celibacy	Self-Nurturance
Cervix	Serial Monogamy
Cohabitation	Trust
Commitment	Pedophilia
Common Law Marriage	Penis
Dysfunctional Family	Perineum
Emotional Availability	Pituitary Gland
Family of Origin	Pornography
Friendship	Premature Ejaculation
Date Rape	Preorgasmic
Dyspareunia	Progesterone
Ejaculation	Proliferatory Phase
Endometrium	Prostate Gland
Epididymus	Rape
Erectile Tissue	Scrotum
Estrogens	Secondary Sex Characteristics
Fallopian Tubes	Semen
Foreskin	Seminal Vesicles
Gender Identity	Sexual Dysfunction
Glans Clitoris	Sexual Harassment
Heterosexuality	Sexual Identity
Homophobia	Sexual Maturity
Homosexuality	Sexual Orientation
Hymen	Testes
Hypothalamus	Testosterone

Impotence
Incest
Intimate Relationships
Labia Majora
Labia Minora
Limerence
Marriage Love
Masturbation
Monogamy

Urethral Opening
Uterus
Vagina
Vaginismus
Variant Sexual Behavior
Vas Deferens
Vasocongestion
Vulva

EXPLORING YOUR ACCESS TO HEALTH

"Are Your Ready For Marriage?"

This inventory is intended to provoke thought about readiness for marriage. For each question respond by indicating "Yes," or "No," or "?" Use the "?" only when you are uncertain. Give each question careful thought. The questionnaire assumes you are considering a specific person as a possible spouse.

1. Even though you may accept advice from your parents, do you make important decisions for yourself? Y

2. Are you often homesick when you are away from home? Y

3. Do you ever feel embarrassed or uneasy in giving or receiving affection? Y

4. Are your feelings easily hurt by criticism? N

5. Do you enjoy working or playing with small children? Y

6. Do you feel embarrassed or uneasy in conversations about sex with older persons or members of the other sex? N

7. Do you have a clear understanding of the physiology of sexual intercourse and reproduction? Y

8. Do you understand the psychological factors determining good sexual adjustment? Y

9. Have you had the experience of using some of your earnings to help meet the expenses of others? Y

10. In an argument, do you lose your temper easily? N

11. Have you and your fiancee ever worked through disagreements to a definite conclusion agreeable to both of you? Y

12. Can you postpone something you want for the sake of later enjoyment? Y

13. Are you normally free from jealousy? Y

14. Have you thought carefully about the goals you will strive for in your marriage? **N**

15. Do you sometimes feel rebellious toward facing the responsibilities of marriage, occupational, or family life? **Y**

16. Have you been able to give up gracefully something you wanted very much? **Y**

17. Do you think of sexual intercourse chiefly as a pleasure experience? **N**

18. Do you find it difficult to differ from others on matters of conduct of dress, even though you disagree with what they think? **N**

19. Do you often have to fight to get your way? **Y**

20. Do you often find yourself making biting remarks or using sarcasm toward others? **N**

21. Do you find yourself strongly emphasizing the glamour aspects of marriage, e.g., the announcement, congratulations, showers, the wedding? **Y**

22. Have you and your fiancee discussed matters which might cause marital conflict? For example: (underline those you have discussed) religious differences; plans for having children; attitudes toward sex; differences in family background; financial arrangement of basic values in life.

Scoring

Record the number of statements to which you responded "NO:" _____. For interpretation and application of your responses to this questionnaire, go to the section entitled "Assessing Health."

Source: Kirkendall, L. A., & Adams, W. J. (1980). *The Students Guide to Marriage and Family Life Literature: An Aid to Individualized Study and Instruction.* Dubuque, IA: Wm. C. Brown. Reprinted by permission.

ASSESSING HEALTH

1. **Readiness For Marriage.** After you have responded to the "Are You Ready for Marriage?" questionnaire, review the items to which you responded "No." An answer of no to questions 2, 3, 4, 6, 10, 15, 18, 19, 20, and 21 and yes to the remainder tends to suggest readiness for marriage. Think about the meaning of your answers and the potential impact on your relationship or future marriage. Perhaps have your potential marriage partner complete the

questionnaire. Discuss the meaning of your answers and how you might avoid potential problems in the relationship.

2. **Developing Intimacy**. Most people would say that "love," "trust," and "honesty," are among the necessary qualities for a lasting, committed, and emotionally intimate relationship. However, for example, the words "I love you" have a rich variety of different meanings for different people. Prepare a list of the qualities you believe are necessary for a committed intimate relationship and/or the characteristics of a desirable relationship partner. Compare your list with the characteristics presented in your textbook. With your partner or friend, discuss the meaning of each quality/characteristic. Explore whether couples tend to assume that each other attaches the same meaning to these attributes. Consider the importance of communicating such meaning in a relationship.

3. **Premarital Contract.** Research your state's codes governing marriage and divorce and also explore your expectations given the possibility of these two events. Review the elements of a premarital contract in your textbook. Based upon the law and your expectations, develop a hypothetical premarital contract. If possible, complete this exercise with your relationship partner.

4. **Your Sexual IQ**. Take a few minutes to complete the "Test Your Sexual IQ" questionnaire in your textbook. Use the questions as a self-test of your knowledge about sexuality. Check your answers and go back to information in the textbook which corresponds to the questions you answered incorrectly.

5. **Reproductive Anatomy and Physiology.** Review the male and female reproductive anatomy and physiology described in your textbook. From memory, label the structure illustrated on the following pages and on a separate sheet of paper, briefly describe the function of each.

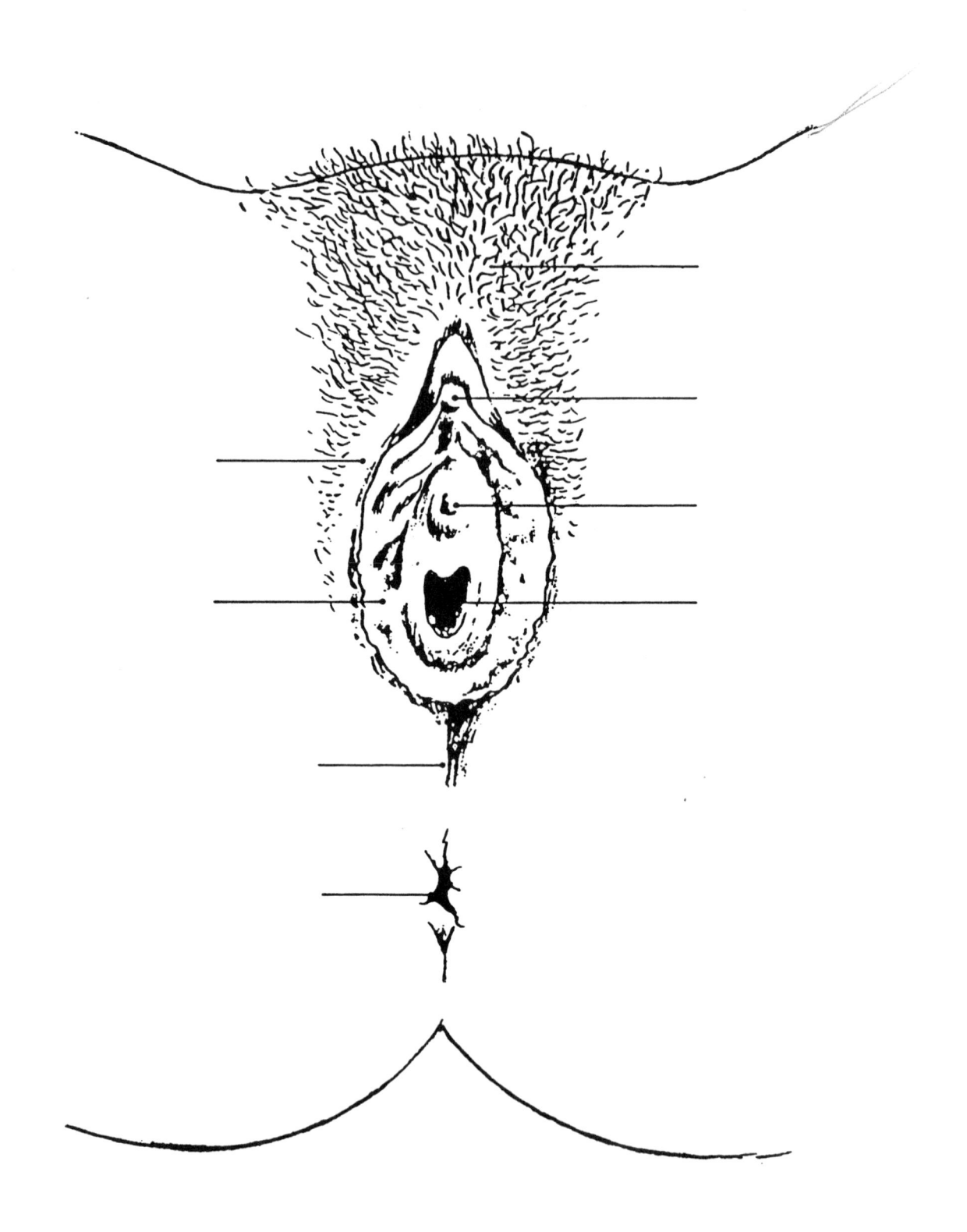

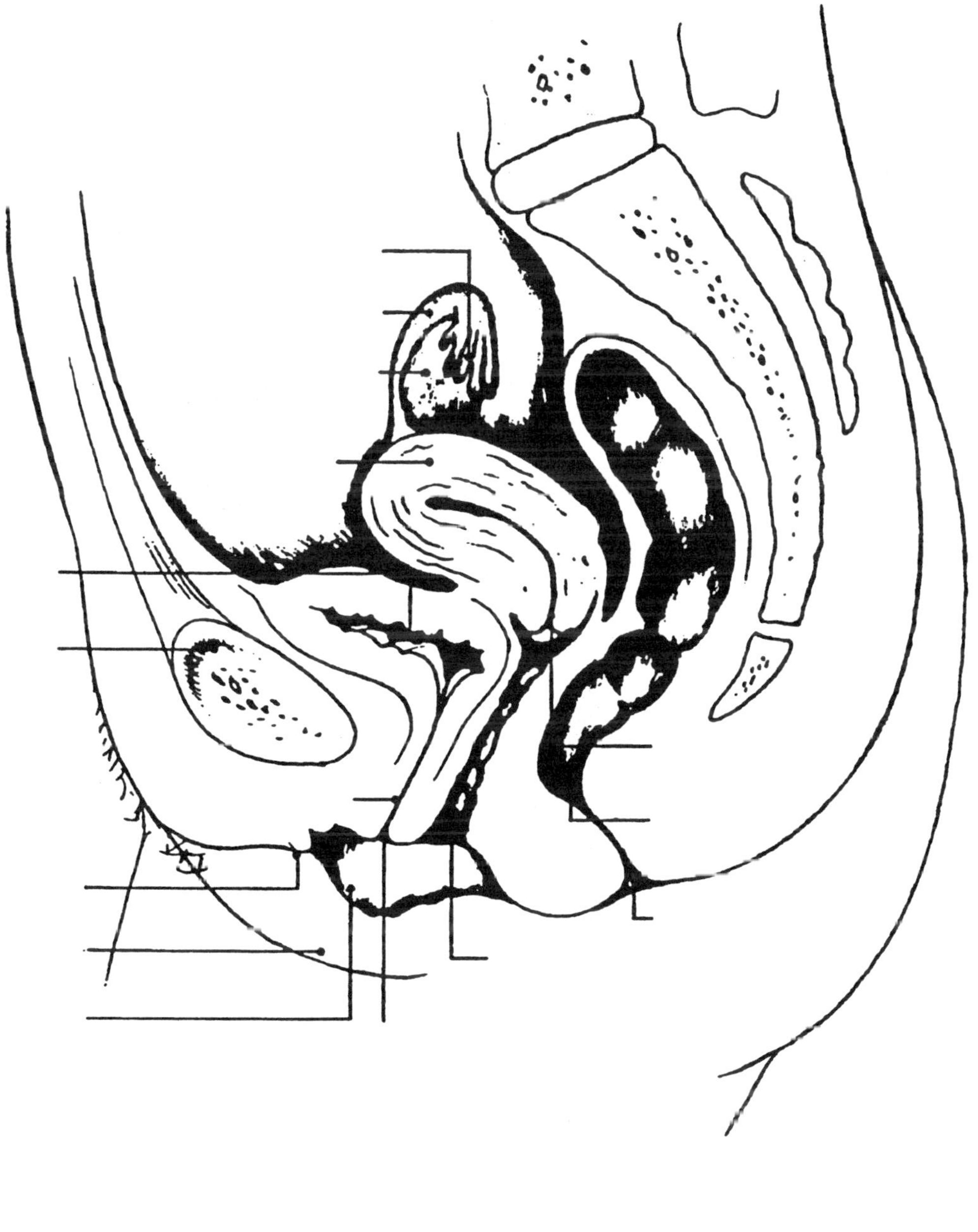

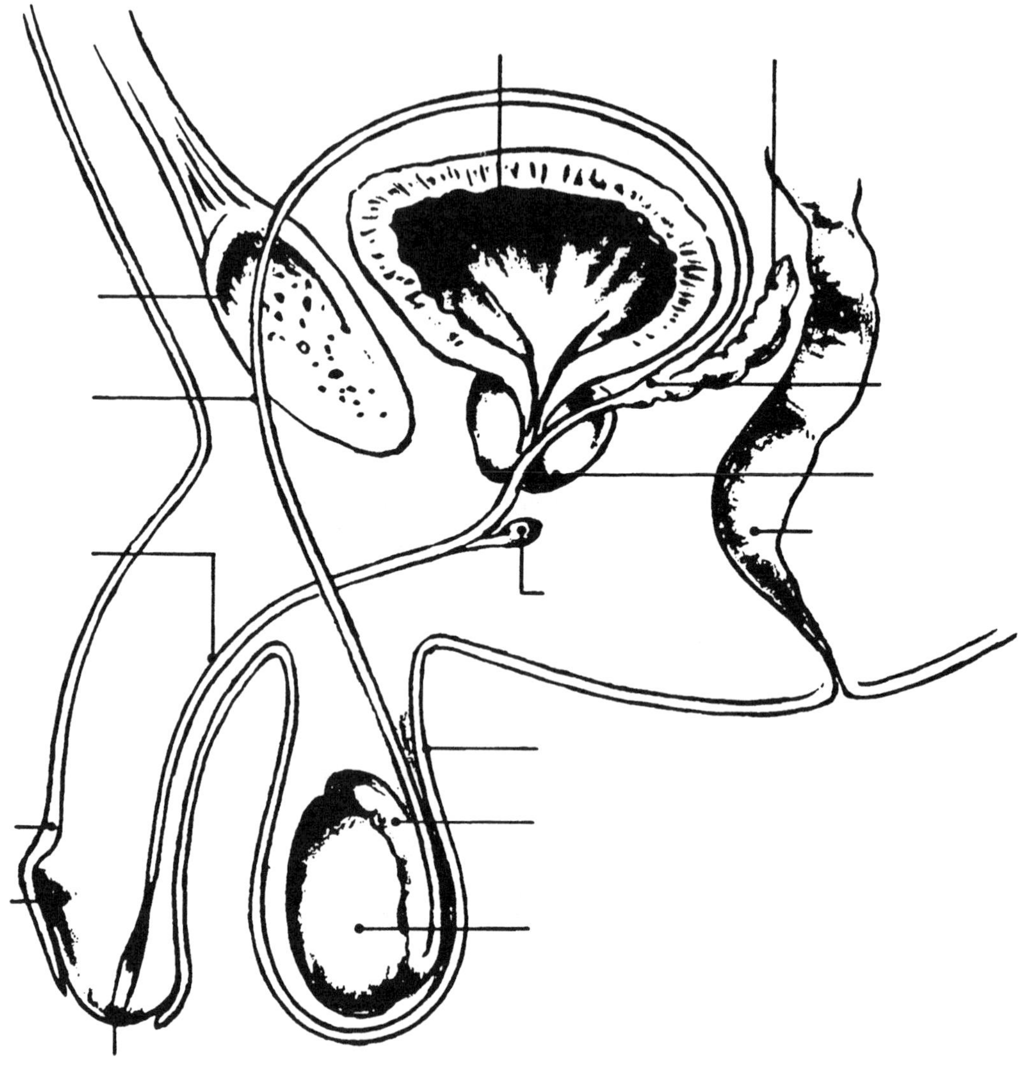

45

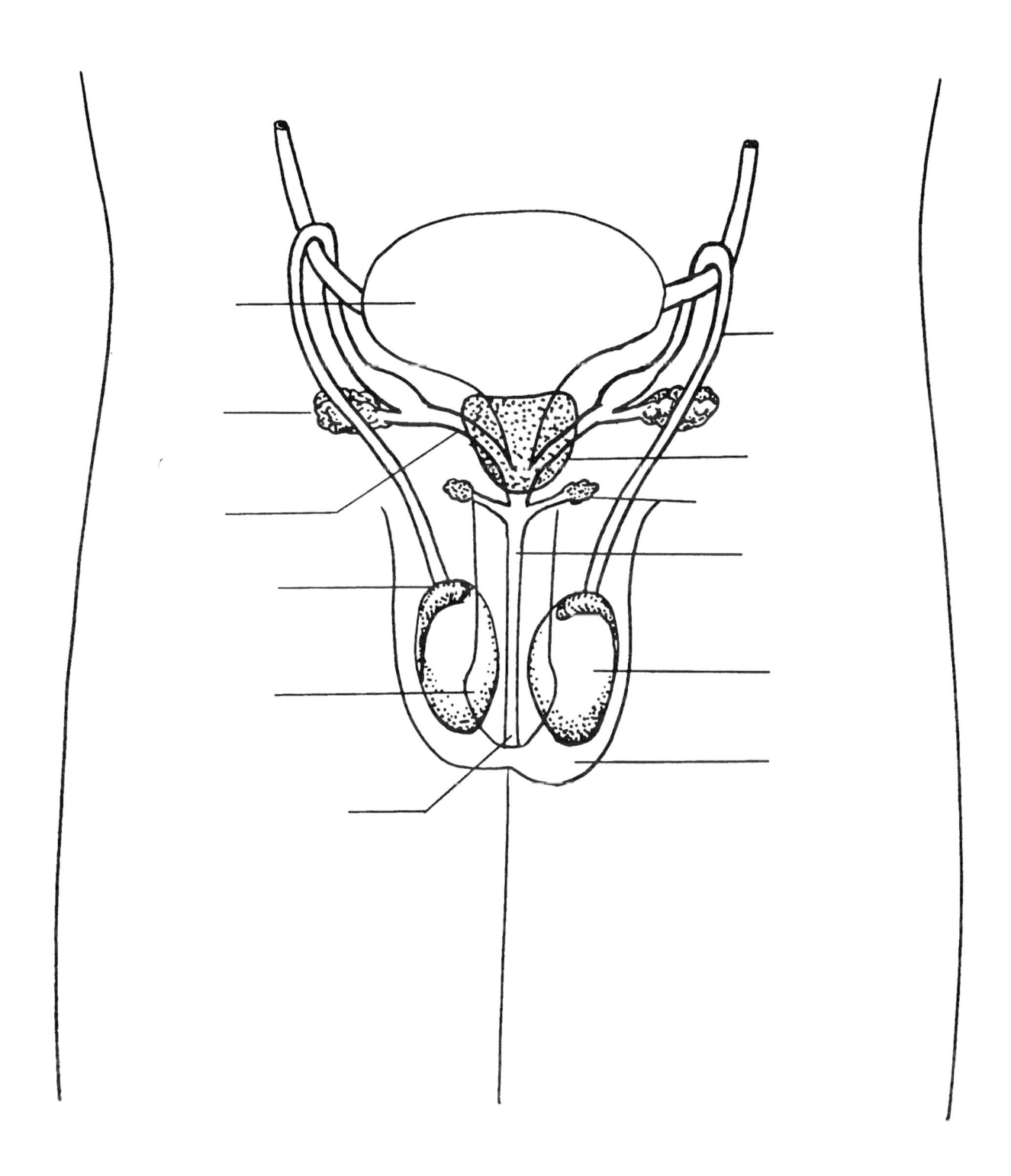

7. **Sexual Attitudes.** Explore your attitudes toward sexuality by completing the following statements. Write the first thing that comes to your mind. Then, go back and think about your responses in greater depth. Do you see a potential for problems arising from any of these attitudes.

Masturbation is _____
_____.

Premarital sexual experiences are _____
_____.

Achieving orgasm is _____
_____.

Having multiple sexual partners is _____
_____.

Initiating the sexual act is _____
_____.

Purchasing contraceptives has to be _____
_____.

Being prepared with a contraceptive is _____
_____.

Calling for a date is _____
_____.

Extramarital sexual experiences are _____
_____.

Homosexuality is _____
_____.

Oral sex is _____
_____.

REVIEW TEST

1. Briefly describe what is meant by an "intimate relationship and list the five types of intimate relationships."

2. Briefly discuss the role of the family as a source of intimacy and dysfunctional relationships.

3. Traditional heterosexual marriage has been characterized as "the social sanctioning of togetherness." From this perspective, what are the advantages of marriage?

4. List five elements of a good relationship.

5. List four warning signs of a declining relationship.

6. List five characteristics of sexually mature people.

7. Briefly discuss the similarities and differences in the sexual responses of males and females.

8. Discuss the various causes of impotence in males and dysparenunia in females.

9. Explain what is meant by the statement: "Good communication skills are essential when confronting problems of sexual ethics."

10. List several measures one can take to protect against rape.

Fill-in-the-Blank

1. Intimacy is developed when _____
   _____
   _____

2. The skills necessary to develop and maintain a good friendship are the same skills that are valuable in developing a committed partnership:
   _____, _____,
   _____, _____,
   and _____.

3. Marriage is legal agreement that involves: _____
   _____, and _____.

4. _____ serve as repositories for the female's developing eggs.

5. Child sexual abuse can be classified as: a) _____
   and (b) _____.

Multiple Choice

1. The ability to give and receive emotionally with another person without fear of being hurt is:
   a. Intimacy
   b. Emotional availability
   c. Self-nurturance
   d. Accountability

2. Adult children of alcoholics:
   a. Are no different from others in their ability to develop and maintain intimate relationships
   b. Have difficulty creating and maintaining intimate relationships
   c. Have little or no problems communicating with their partners
   d. Have the necessary skills to development a healthy relationship

3. The degree of confidence felt in a relationship is:
   a. Trust
   b. Dependability
   c. Faith
   d. None of the above

4. Factors that contribute to the development of a healthy relationship include all of the following, except:
   a. Trust
   b. Communication
   c. Sense of humor
   d. Sexual satisfaction

5. Breakdowns in relationships usually begin with:
   a. Unresolved conflicts
   b. Changes in communication
   c. Sexual difficulties
   d. Spending time apart

6. Sexuality identity is defined by a person's:
   a. Sexual gender
   b. Sexual preference
   c. Body image
   d. All of the above

7. The hollow, muscular tube through which menstrual flow leaves the female's body is:
   a. Fallopian tubes
   b. Vagina
   c. Uterus
   d. Cervix

8. Testes are responsible for the production of:
   a. Progestin
   b. Follicle stimulating hormone
   c. Testosterone
   d. Androgens

9. People who are attracted to and prefer sexual activity with people of both sexes are:
   a. Heterosexual
   b. Homosexual
   c. Bisexual
   d. Homogeneous

10. The inability to attain or maintain an erection or sufficient penile rigidity for intercourse is called:
    a. Erectile difficulties
    b. Premature ejaculation
    c. Impotence
    d. Performance anxiety

CHAPTER 5

PREGNANCY, CHILDBIRTH, AND BIRTH CONTROL

CHAPTER OVERVIEW

The decision to become a parent has become a choice which is influenced by many factors. The responsibilities to have a child include more than financial obligations. Parents must also provide a loving and nurturing environment that provides for the emotional, social, and spiritual needs of their child. Once the decision is made to have children, a successful pregnancy involves a healthy environment in which a the baby develops. Chapter 5 explores the issues concerning pregnancy, childbirth, and parenting before deciding to conceive. Today's knowledge and technology also allow individuals the choice not to have children. Thus, choosing an effective method of birth control that will prevent pregnancy is a serious consideration. Chapter 5 discusses the two categories of contraceptive methods and explores the advantages and disadvantages of each method. Chapter 5 also familiarizes you with the practical, scientific, and philosophical considerations associated with such issues as abortion, infertility, and surrogate motherhood.

LEARNING OBJECTIVES

Upon completion of Chapter 5 you should be able to:

1. Discuss the considerations in deciding to have a child.
2. List and discuss the issues to consider for a successful pregnancy, i.e., drugs, X-rays, nutrition, environmental exposures, immunization, practitioner, and maternal age.
3. Describe the process of pregnancy with particular attention to the signs of pregnancy, fetal development, and the three trimesters of gestation.
4. List and describe the methods available for prenatal testing and screening.
5. Describe labor and delivery.
6. List and briefly describe the various birth alternatives.
7. Explain the importance of "colostrum" for the newborn.
8. Describe the circumstances where C-section and VBAC would be indicated.
9. List and briefly describe the various reasons for pregnancy loss.
10. List the conditions which are necessary for conception.
11. List and briefly describe how each of the two categories of contraceptives acts to prevent pregnancy.
12. List and briefly describe the different forms of contraceptives with attention to their use, action in preventing pregnancy, effectiveness, advantages, and disadvantages.
13. Describe the provisions of the Supreme Court decision in "Roe v. Wade."

14. List and describe the available methods of abortion, at what points in pregnancy each may be indicated, and their associated risks and complications.
15. List and discuss the reasons for infertility and the available solutions/alternatives.
16. Describe the issues surrounding surrogate motherhood.

KEY TERMS

Abortion
Afterbirth
Alternative Insemination
Amniocentesis
Body Temperature Method
Calendar Method
Cerebral Palsy
Cervical Cap
Cervical Mucus Method
Cesarean Section
Cloning
Conception
Condom
Contraception
Contraceptive Sponge
Dilation and Evacuation (D&E)
Diaphragm
Down's Syndrome
Ectopic Pregnancy
Embryo
Embryo Freezing
Embryo Transfer
Endometriosis
Female Condom

Fertility Drugs
Fetal Alcohol Syndrome
Fetus
Induction Abortion
In Vitro Fertilization
Low Sperm Count
Miscarriage
Morning-after Pill
Natural Method
Nonsurgical Embryo Transfer
Oral Contraceptives
Placenta
Pelvic Inflammatory Disease
Rh Factor
Spermicide
Sterilization
Stillbirth
Teratogenic
Toxic Shock Syndrome
Trimester
Vacuum Aspiration
Vasectomy
Withdrawal

EXPLORING YOUR ACCESS TO HEALTH

"Baby Costs"

No one would want to put a dollar value on the worth of a child; however, certain costs cannot be avoided. Sometimes choices need to be made between items that cannot all be afforded. Sometimes there are ways to minimize the costs.

Directions:

A. For each item below, first determine and label each item as (N) necessary to pay for, (U) unnecessary to have, (B) could be borrowed, (F) free, (I) covered by insurance, (L) the number could be limited to less than stated.
B. Use ads, catalogs, phone calls, store visits, advice of people with young children, and other references to determine the cost of those items it would be necessary to pay for.

Item to Consider	Rating	Cost	Item to Consider	Rating	Cost
Prenatal Care	_____	_____	2 4-oz. Bottles with Nipples	_____	_____
Maternity Clothing	_____	_____	1 Bottle Brush	_____	_____
Prenatal Classes	_____	_____	Baby Soap	_____	_____
Delivery	_____	_____	Baby Oil	_____	_____
4 - 6 dozen Diapers	_____	_____	Baby Powder	_____	_____
Diaper Service (1 yr.)	_____	_____	Baby Shampoo	_____	_____
Disposable Diapers (1 yr. - about 85 boxes)	_____	_____	Rectal Thermometer	_____	_____
4 - 6 Knit Shirts	_____	_____	Petroleum Jelly	_____	_____
6 Knit Sleepers	_____	_____	Pediatrician	_____	_____
2 - 3 Sleeping Bags	_____	_____	Formula (1 yr.)	_____	_____
2 Sweater Sets	_____	_____	Toys	_____	_____
Rubber Pants (4 pr.)	_____	_____	Baby Pictures	_____	_____
4 Plastic-Backed Bibs	_____	_____	Nursery Decorations	_____	_____
4 Crib Sheets	_____	_____	Babysitter	_____	_____
3 Waterproof Crib Sheets	_____	_____	Laundry Costs (wash & dry plus detergent & softener)	_____	_____
1 Pkg. Waterproof Pads for Crib or Lap	_____	_____	Wind-up Swing	_____	_____
4 Light Blankets	_____	_____	Scale	_____	_____
1 Warm Blanket	_____	_____	Changing Table	_____	_____
2 Washcloths	_____	_____	Crib and Mattress and Bumpers	_____	_____
2 Hand Towels	_____	_____	Car Seat	_____	_____
2 Bath Towels	_____	_____	Playpen	_____	_____
Highchair	_____	_____	Vaporizer	_____	_____
Infant Seat	_____	_____	Feeding Dish	_____	_____
Stroller	_____	_____	Bathtub	_____	_____
Diaper Bag	_____	_____	Food (1 yr.)	_____	_____
6-8 8-oz. Bottles with Nipples	_____	_____	**Total**		_____

C. Total your costs and go to the section entitled "Baby Costs" for the meaning and interpretation of your score.

Source: Kentucky Department of Education (1991), *Parenting and Family Life Skills Education Curriculum.* Used with permission of author.

"Personal Contraceptive Assessment"

For each of the following contraceptive methods, note the effectiveness, advantages, disadvantages, how comfortable you and your partner would feel using the approach, and the likelihood you would use it consistently without error.

Method	Effectiveness	Advantages	Disadvantages	Comfort	Would Use Consistently Without Error
Condom					
Foams, Jellies, & Creams					
Diaphragm with Cream or Jelly					
Sponge					
Cervical Cap					
Condom plus Spermicide					
Contraceptive Pill					
Rhythm: Mucus BBT Calendar					
Progestasert-T					
Sterilization					

ASSESSING HEALTH

1. **Readiness for Parenting.** Complete the "Am I Parent Material" questionnaire in your textbook with your partner. After reviewing your responses, consider the reasons for these attitudes, how they could be modified to more mature perspectives, and restate them below. Think about the effects of "self-talk" on attitudes and behavior and how these new statements could be used to increase your readiness to parent.

2. **Baby Costs.** After researching the costs of a child during the first year, do you feel that you are financially ready to raise a child? What would be some of the other less tangible costs that would be associated with having a child? This total cost is just for one year. How much do you think it would cost to raise a child to adulthood? What sacrifices would you and your partner need to make to raise a child?

3. **Contraceptive Awareness.** Review your responses to the "Personal Contraceptive Assessment." If appropriate, evaluate the various considerations in choosing a contraceptive with your relationship partner. Keep in mind that the "best" and "most effective" contraceptive method is the one you will use most consistently and accurately.

4. **Visitation.** The actions we take to affect our reproductive health should be those of informed choice. There are a variety of community agencies and programs which serve different aspects of reproductive health and welcome inquiries. Plan a visit to one of these programs, i.e., Family Planning or Planned Parenthood Center, Birthing center, prepared childbirth program, La Leache League, etc. Before your visit, formulate questions of interest. After the visit, write a summary of your findings.

REVIEW TEST

Short Answer

1. List the considerations in deciding to have a child.

2. List and describe the methods available for prenatal testing and screening.

3. Discuss the issues to consider for a successful pregnancy.

4. Describe labor and delivery.

5. Briefly describe the various reasons for pregnancy loss.

6. List the available methods of abortion. At what point in pregnancy may each be indicated? What are their associated risks and complications?

7. Discuss the reasons for infertility and available solutions/alternatives.

8. Discuss the issues surrounding surrogate motherhood.

9. Describe the provisions of the Supreme Court decision in "Roe vs. Wade." List the issues surrounding abortion that have contributed to this decision and its controversy.

10. List and briefly describe the various birth alternatives.

Fill-in-the-Blank

1. In the _____ trimester the fetus is particularly susceptible to the teratogenic effects of certain chemical substances.

2. The birth defect which is most common among babies born to mothers older than 35 is called _____ _____.

3. The procedure that uses high frequency sound waves to determine the size and position of the fetus is called _____.

4. Contraceptive methods can be categorized as _____ methods, such as condoms, and _____ methods, such as tubal ligation and vasectomy.

5. The most common reason for infertility among men is _____ _____.

Multiple Choice

1. Modern pregnancy tests are designed to detect the presence of:
   a. FSH
   b. LH
   c. HCG
   d. RU-486

2. The typical time period for a full-term human pregnancy is in the range of:
   a. 150-175 days
   b. 175-200 days
   c. 240-300 days
   d. 365-400 days

3. A fertilized egg from conception until the end of two months development is called an:
   a. Embryo
   b. Zygote
   c. Fetus
   d. Ova

4. Detection of major health defects in a fetus as early as the fourteenth to eighteenth weeks of pregnancy is performed by:
   a. Ultrasound
   b. Fetoscopy
   c. Amniocentesis
   d. Sonography

5. A central nervous system disorder characterized by uncontrolled muscle spasms that can result from lack of oxygen at birth is called:
   a. Cerebral palsy
   b. Muscular dystrophy
   c. Multiple sclerosis
   d. Hemophilia

6. Postpartum depression is characterized by:
   a. Energy depletion
   b. Anxiety
   c. Mood swings
   d. All of the above

7. A chemical substance that kills sperm in known as:
   a. Spermatogenesis
   b. Sperm barrier
   c. Spermicide
   d. All of the above

8. Most oral contraceptives contain a combination of:
   a. Follicle stimulating hormone and progesterone
   b. Estrogen and progesterone
   c. Estrogen and luteinizing hormone
   d. Follicle stimulating hormone and luteinizing hormone

9. A T-shaped plastic device that is implanted in the uterus to prevent conception is:
   a. Cervical sponge
   b. Diaphragm
   c. Vaginal Ring
   d. Intrauterine device

10. The most commonly used method of first trimester abortion is:
    a. RU-486
    b. Vacuum aspiration
    c. Dilation and evacuation
    d. Dilation and curettage

CHAPTER 6

NUTRITION: EATING FOR OPTIMAL HEALTH

CHAPTER OVERVIEW

Nutrition plays a vital lifestyle role in enhancing all the dimensions of human well-being. With an overabundance of food and food choices, Americans should have fewer nutritional problems. However, Americans suffer from such nutritionally related diseases as heart disease, certain types of cancer, hypertension, cirrhosis of the liver, tooth decay, and chronic obesity. Eating for optimal health means consuming a diet that is properly balanced in calories and nutrients to maximize health and reduce risk to disease. Chapter 6 presents a comprehensive examination of the relationship between nutrition and health and offers specific guidelines to assist in maintaining a healthful diet. The six nutrients and their role in body function are examined and recommended food sources are provided. Further, Chapter 6 examines alternative nutritional choices, including vegetarian diets, fast foods, and eating on a student budget.

LEARNING OBJECTIVES

Upon completion of Chapter 6 you should be able to:

1. Differentiate between hunger and appetite.
2. Describe the factors that influence eating habits.
3. Explain what is meant by "diets of affluence" and their consequences for Americans.
4. Describe the average American diet and its associated problems.
5. List the Dietary Goals for the U.S. and the Dietary Guidelines for Americans.
6. Describe the digestive process and its role in maintaining proper nutrition.
7. List and describe the basic nutrients. Give particular attention to their sources and function in health and disease.
8. List the four basic food groups and describe the "fifth food group."
9. Differentiate between the three major types of vegetarian diets.
10. Describe the healthy and unhealthy aspects of fast foods.
11. Recommend ways one can maintain a nutritious diet within the confines of student life.

KEY TERMS

Amino Acids	Incomplete Protein
Anemia	LDLs

Appetite	Macrominerals
Calorie	Monosaccharides
Carbohydrates	Plaque
Cellulose	Polysaccharides
Cholesterol	Proteins
Complex Carbohydrates	RDAs
Complete Protein	Saliva
Dehydration	Saturated Fats
Digestive Process	Simple Sugars
Disaccharides	Small Intestine
Esophagus	Stomach
Essential Amino Acids	Trace Minerals
Fats	Triglyceride
Glycogen	Unsaturated Fats
HDLs	Vegetarianism
Hunger	Vitamins
Hypervitaminosis	

EXPLORING YOUR ACCESS TO HEALTH

"Daily Food Diary"

Keep a record of your daily food intake for one week. Make a copy of this recording sheet and carry it with you, noting the foods you eat as you eat them. Later, conduct a basic analysis of the nutritional value of your diet, considering the portion sizes, calories, food groups, and nutrients consumed.

Food & Source	Portion Size	Food Group	Nutrients
Day 1			
Day 2			

Day 3

Day 4

Day 5

Day 6

Day 7

"Dietary Guidelines for Americans"

For each of the following guidelines, write a statement which reflects an evaluation of your dietary behavior. Use your "Daily Food Diary" and information in your textbook to assist in completing this evaluation.

1. Eat a variety of foods, including fruits, vegetables, whole grains, enriched breads, cereals, and grain products; milk, cheese, and yogurt; meats, poultry, fish, and eggs; legumes (dried peas and beans).

2. Maintain ideal weight (see Chapter 7).

3. Avoid too much fat, saturated fat, and cholesterol (although excluded from the 1985 guidelines, this remains an important recommendation).

4. Eat foods with adequate starch and fiber.

5. Avoid too much sugar.

6. Avoid too much sodium.

7. If you drink alcohol, do so in moderation.

Source: U.S. Department of Agriculture, *Nutrition and Your Health: Dietary Guidelines for Americans.* (Washington, D.C., U.S. Government Printing Office. 1980).

ASSESSING HEALTH

1. **Daily Food Diary.** Complete the "Daily Food Diary" and analyze the nutritional value of your diet according to calories, food groups, and nutrient content. Summarize the results of your analysis below. These findings may form the basis for a real self-change project to improve your nutrition (see Chapter 1).

2. **Dietary Guidelines.** After completing the "Dietary Guidelines for Americans" evaluation, summarize the results below and indicate specific changes you need to make in achieving the U.S. Dietary Goals presented in Table 13.2 in your textbook. Consider your findings from this and the previous exercise as the basis of a self-change project (see Chapter 1).

3. **Fast Food Analysis.** Eat at one or more fast food restaurants and then evaluate the caloric and nutrient value of each meal (nutritional information is usually available upon request). From the analysis, does it appear that the restaurants you evaluated are responding to consumer demands by providing more nutritionally sound food choices (see your textbook)?

4. **Comparison Shopping.** Visit a local supermarket and health food store to compare the prices of some standard food items (nuts, raisins, mixed dried fruit, desserts, etc.). Evaluate the cost versus food value of the items from the two sources and summarize your findings below. Are there real differences in food value which would justify variations in prices?

5. **Food Label Analysis.** Below, record the ingredients from the labels of several of your favorite foods. Note which ingredients comprise the greatest proportion of the product (labeled in descending order) and the sugar, sodium, cholesterol, and saturated fat content; and make general statements about the healthfulness of these foods.

REVIEW TEST

Short Answer

1. List and briefly describe the six basic nutrients.

2. Briefly describe the three types of vegetarian diets.

3. Briefly explain how some fast food chains have begun to respond to consumer demands.

4. List four steps students can take to maintain a nutritious diet within the confines of a restrictive budget.

5. Describe the factors that influence eating habits.

6. List the Dietary Goals for the U.S. and the Dietary Guidelines for Americans.

7. List the four basic food groups and describe the "fifth" food group.

8. Describe the average American Diet and its associated problems.

9. Differentiate between hunger and appetite.

10. Explain what is meant by "diets of affluence" and their consequences for Americans.

Fill-in-the-Blank

1. Our _____ is stimulated when we want to eat something because it looks or smells good.

2. The building blocks of proteins that the adult body cannot synthesize in adequate amounts are referred to as _____ _____ _____.

3. Vitamins are classified as either _____ _____ or _____ _____.

4. Diets that are deficient in _____ may result in symptoms such as bleeding gums and muscle weakness.

5. _____ are inorganic, indestructible elements that aid physiological processes within the body.

Multiple Choice

1. A unit of measure that indicates the amount of energy obtained from a particular food is called a:
   a. Amino acid
   b. Carbohydrate
   c. Calorie
   d. Vitamin

2. The process by which foods are broken down and either absorbed or excreted by the body is known as:
   a. Digestive process
   b. Elimination process
   c. Metabolism process
   d. Nutritional process

3. Which of the following is a key dietary recommendation in *the Surgeon General's Report on Nutrition and Health* ?
   a. Increase consumption of fat and cholesterol
   b. Increase sodium intake
   c. Decrease consumption of complex carbohydrates and fiber
   d. Achieve and maintain a desirable body weight by balancing calorie intake with energy expenditure

4. Substances that are made up of amino acids that are major components of cells are:
   a. Water
   b. Carbohydrates
   c. Proteins
   d. Minerals

5. Amino acids that the body cannot synthesize in adequate amounts are referred to as:
   a. Nonessential amino acids
   b. Essential amino acids
   c. Complete amino acids
   d. Incomplete amino acids

6. Fats:
   a. Are vital in the maintenance of healthy skin and hair
   b. Are vital for insulation of the body organs against shock
   c. Are vital for maintenance of body temperature
   d. All of the above

7. A major cause of atherosclerosis is:
   a. Plaque
   b. High density lipoproteins
   c. Unsaturated fats
   d. Monounsaturated fats

8. Inorganic, indestructible elements that aid physiological processes within the body are:
   a. Vitamins
   b. Amino acids
   c. Minerals
   d. High density lipoproteins

9. The four basic food groups include all of the following except:
   a. Milk and milk products
   b. Meat and meat alternatives
   c. Alcohol
   d. Fruits and vegetables

10. The major energy suppliers of the body are:
    a. Vitamins
    b. Carbohydrates
    c. Proteins
    d. Minerals

CHAPTER 7

MANAGING YOUR WEIGHT: CONSUMING AND EXPENDING ENERGY

CHAPTER OVERVIEW

Maintaining reasonable body weight can provide numerous health-enhancing benefits. Yet, for many, managing weight is a tremendous challenge. The American obsession with thinness has turned being overweight into a social and emotional problem, both in cause and effect. We are offered a myriad of approaches to dieting and extensive amounts of misinformation about weight control. In Chapter 7 you are acquainted with the facts and fallacies about body weight and techniques for assessing body fat. Furthermore, Chapter 7 describes the factors that determine obesity, including heredity, hunger and appetite, developmental factors, endocrine influences, psychosocial factors, metabolic changes, pregnancy, and lack of physical activity. Finally, techniques for weight reduction and healthful approaches to weight management are discussed.

LEARNING OBJECTIVES

Upon completion of Chapter 7 you should be able to:

1. Discuss the reasons for the American obsession with thinness and the relationship between body weight and health.
2. Describe the consequences of being below an acceptable minimum level of body fat.
3. Discuss the problems of anorexia nervosa and bulimia in terms of cause, symptoms and signs, treatment, and prognosis.
4. Describe the normal ranges of body fat for men and women and explain why they differ.
5. Describe the various methods of determining ideal weight and body fat.
6. Discuss the factors which contribute to body weight/obesity.
7. Differentiate between weight loss plans that are sound and those that are not recommended.
8. List and describe the "strategies to ensure success" in losing weight.
9. Discuss the steps in changing eating behavior.

KEY TERMS

Adaptive Thermogenesis
Anorexia Nervosa
Appetite
Basal Metabolic Rate (BMR)

Hyperplasia
Hypertrophy
Nutrition/Exercise Training
Obesity

BIA
Body Mass Index
Brown Fat Cells
Bulimia
Girth and Circumference Measures
Exercise Metabolic Rate (EMR)
Hunger
Hydrostatic Weighing

Pinch Test
Plateau
Resting Metabolic Rate (RMR)
Set-Point Theory
Skin-Fold Caliper Test
Soft-Tissue Roentgenogram
Thyroid Gland
TOBEC

EXPLORING YOUR ACCESS TO HEALTH

"Your Emotional Investment in Eating"

To evaluate the contribution of emotions to your eating habits, use the following descriptions and circle the number next to each statement that best describes you.

---

0 = Never; total avoidance
1 = Seldom; about 1% to 3% of the time or from 4 times yearly to once a month.
2 = Occasionally; about 10% of the time or 2 to 3 times a month.
3 = Often; about 20% to 50% of the time or 1 to 3 times a week.
4 = Very frequently; about 50% to 90% of the time or as much as every other day to every day.

1.	Eat excessively when bored or depressed.	0	1	2	3	4
2.	Eat when suffering from insomnia.	0	1	2	3	4
3.	Eat foods you know are "bad" for you.	0	1	2	3	4
4.	Prefer eating alone.	0	1	2	3	4
5.	Feel conspicuous or embarrassed when eating with others.	0	1	2	3	4
6.	Parents used, made available, or encouraged sweets.	0	1	2	3	4
7.	Fear weight gain.	0	1	2	3	4
8.	"Hell with it all" feeling.	0	1	2	3	4
9.	Will sneak or hide foods.	0	1	2	3	4
10.	Use alcoholic beverages.	0	1	2	3	4
11.	Eat foods discouraged by parents.	0	1	2	3	4
12.	Eat or drink in secrecy.	0	1	2	3	4
13.	Use drugs (tranquilizers, sleeping pills, appetite suppressants, etc.).	0	1	2	3	4
14.	Self-conscious of how my body looks.	0	1	2	3	4
15.	I mistreat myself.	0	1	2	3	4
16.	Wish I looked different.	0	1	2	3	4
17.	Feelings of being in the midst of "struggle" (over diet or otherwise).	0	1	2	3	4
18.	Waves of anger or hostility.	0	1	2	3	4

19. Feelings (over diet or other factor) of
    being "rushed" or sense of time urgency.   0   1   2   3   4
20. Fatigue or "wiped out" feelings.   0   1   2   3   4
21. Uncontrollable hunger urges.   0   1   2   3   4
22. Gulp my food.   0   1   2   3   4
23. Stuff myself.   0   1   2   3   4
24. Indulge in sweets.   0   1   2   3   4
25. Eat when not hungry.   0   1   2   3   4
26. Eat and run.   0   1   2   3   4
27. Cravings for sweets.   0   1   2   3   4
28. Meals or heavy snack after 7 PM.   0   1   2   3   4
29. Eating within an hour of retiring.   0   1   2   3   4
30. Eating binges.   0   1   2   3   4

Total Score   _____

Scoring

Add the numbers you circled and enter your total score. Go to the "Emotions and Eating" exercise in the next section to learn more about the meaning and application of your score.

ASSESSING HEALTH

1. **Your Calorie Requirements.** The following exercise gives you general guidelines to use in calculating your caloric requirements for maintaining and losing weight.

   To Maintain Your Weight:

   a. Take the midpoint of the desirable weight range of your sex, height, and body type from Table 7.1 in your textbook. (If you are a man of medium frame who is 5'10" tall, for example, take the midpoint of the range 151-163, or 157). Enter that number at the right.

                                                                  _____

   b. If you are female, multiply this number by 16; if you are male, multiply it by 18.

                                                              x _____

   This number represents the approximate number of calories you need per day for rest and light activity.

                                                              = _____

   c. Add from Table 7.3 in your textbook the average number of calories you expend per day in moderate or vigorous activity. If, for instance, you walk at a moderate rate for an hour a day but do little other exercise, add 345 calories.

+ _____

This number represents your approximate daily maintenance-level calorie requirement. If you are gaining weight, you are likely consuming more than this number of calories.

_____

To Lose One Pound a Week:

Subtract 500 calories from maintenance calories:

_____ maintenance calories.

____-500____

_____

Source : J. LaPlace, *Health.* (Englewood Cliffs, NJ: Prentice Hall, 1987), 139.

2. **Emotions and Eating.** After completing the "Emotional Investment in Eating" inventory, find the meaning of your score in the following guide.

   A score of 60 or below suggests that you have a good relationship with your body and that you are sensitive to your physical needs.

   Scores of 60 -80 are in the average range for normally healthy people.

   Scoring between 81 and 95 suggests that your eating is, to some extent, too emotionally connected.

   A score of 96 or above indicates excessive emotional influences on your eating behaviors.

   If you scored 81 or above, identify the statements on the inventory which appear to have contributed most to your high score. Also, review the discussions of "psychological factors" which contribute to weight problems and "changing your eating behavior" in your textbook. Consider how the factors you identified act to direct or "trigger" your eating and how you will use this information to modify your eating behavior.

3. **Self-Observation.** As you learned from the "Health Behavior Change" exercise in Chapter 1 of this workbook, self-directing behavior requires self-knowledge. After completing the "Eating Behaviors Record," examine your entries to identify your eating patterns, the factors which tend to trigger and support your eating behaviors, and the ways you expend the calories consumed Also, note any changes in body weight revealed on your graph. Typically, self-observation in itself will result in some behavior change without any overt effort to change one's behavior. Below, summarize your

findings and how you could apply this information to managing your eating behaviors and body weight.

4. **Body Composition.** Contact the Wellness Program, Student Health Service, or Physical Education Department at your school about body fat determination. Your instructor may be helpful in arranging for this measurement. Compare your findings with the normal ranges of body fat presented in your textbook. It also will be interesting to compare results with the ideal weight determinations for your height, frame, and sex given in your textbook.

5. **Weight-Management Plan.** Use the information from the preceding exercises and the principles presented in your textbook and Chapter 1 of this workbook in developing a self-change plan to modify or maintain your body weight/composition.

REVIEW TEST

Short Answer

1. Briefly discuss the reasons for America's obsession with thinness.

2. List the health risks associated with excessive body weight.

3. Briefly describe the concept of adaptive thermogenesis.

4. Briefly describe the importance of endocrine influence in most obesity.

5. Briefly describe the eating pattern and activity level of the majority of overweight people.

6. We know that weight-loss efforts that work for one person do not necessarily work for another. Briefly describe what most successful weight-loss efforts must consider.

7. List 5 strategies to ensure success in losing weight.

8. Give 3 examples of removing triggers or substituting behaviors to help in developing more sensible eating patterns.

9. Briefly describe the various methods of determining ideal weight and body fat.

10. Discuss the problems of anorexia nervosa and bulemia in terms of their cause, symptoms and signs, treatment, and prognosis.

Fill-in-the-Blank

1. Among the most reliable height-weight guides is the _____ _____.

2. _____ _____ is an eating disorder characterized by an almost psychotic obsession with thinness.

3. The amount of energy used at complete rest is known as the _____ _____ _____.

4. One pound of body fat contains approximately _____ kcal.

5. _____/_____ _____ involves teaching a person to eat and exercise responsibly.

Multiple Choice

1. The ability to lose weight includes which of the following factors?
   a. Genetic predisposition
   b. Hormonal imbalances
   c. Beliefs
   d. All of the above

2. An accumulation of fat beyond what is considered normal for a person's age, sex, and body type is called:
   a. Body composition
   b. Obesity
   c. Overweight
   d. Body fat

3. Excessively low fat in females may lead to:
   a. Hyperthermia
   b. Dysmenorrhea
   c. Amenorrhea
   d. Endometriosis

4. An inborn physiological response to nutritional needs is:
   a. Hunger
   b. Appetite
   c. Satiety
   d. Adaptive thermogenesis

5. According to theories of hyperplasia:
   a. The number of fat cells decrease with weight loss
   b. The number of fat cells remain constant but their size decreases with weight loss
   c. The number of fat cells increase with weight loss
   d. None of the above

6. The amount of energy used at complete rest is:
   a. Exercise metabolic rate
   b. Resting metabolic rate
   c. Basal metabolic rate
   d. Nuritional metabolic rate

7. The best way to improve one's chance for long-term success with weight loss is:
   a. Nutrition/Exercise training
   b. Liposuction
   c. Cambridge diet
   d. Liquid diets

8. The major cause of low activity levels is:
   a. Vacuum cleaners
   b. Automobiles
   c. TV remote controls
   d. All of the above

9. Fat that is necessary for normal physiological functioning is called:
   a. Body fat
   b. Essential fat
   c. Brown fat
   d. Storage fat

10. The gland that is located in the throat that produces a hormone that regulates metabolism is the:
    a. Lymph gland
    b. Thyroid gland
    c. Adrenal gland
    d. Pancreas

CHAPTER 8

AEROBIC EXERCISE FOR FITNESS AND HEALTH

CHAPTER OVERVIEW

Americans are constantly exposed to information about the benefits of physical fitness. The accumulated body of research clearly suggests that regular exercise can dramatically enhance physical, mental, and social well-being. Aerobic activity at moderate intensities may be the best kind of exercise to improve health status. Chapter 8 compares the two types of exercise (anaerobic and aerobic exercise) and describes the energy sources that fuel these activities. Aerobic exercise has several benefits, including increased cardiovascular fitness, metabolic alterations, improved psychological well-being and productivity. Chapter 8 further discusses the importance of intensity and duration for maximizing the cardiovascular benefits of aerobic exercise. While aerobic activities have many positive benefits, care should be taken to reduce the dangerous effects that hot and cold weather may have on exercise. Finally, Chapter 8 explores the numerous types of aerobic exercise, their advantages and disadvantages, as well as their special considerations.

LEARNING OBJECTIVES

Upon completion of Chapter 8 you should be able to:

1. Describe the benefits of cardiovascular fitness.
2. Differentiate between anaerobic and aerobic exercise.
3. Compare fast-twitch and slow-twitch muscle fibers.
4. Identify the primary energy sources for muscle fuel for exercise.
5. Identify the two factors that are critical for energy utilization.
6. List at least five benefits of aerobic exercise.
7. Describe detraining and its effects on maintaining fitness.
8. List several principles to consider when initiating a conditioning program.
9. Describe the effects of catecholamines that are released during exercise.
10. Determine your target heart rate.
11. Describe the various methods of monitoring exercise intensity.
12. Describe the importance of determining exercise duration.
13. Discuss exercise adherence and the factors that contribute to comfortable exercise.
14. Describe the dangers of exercising in hot and cold weather.
15. Compare and contrast the various types of aerobic activities, including the advantages and disadvantages of each type, and special considerations.
16. Discuss the benefits of healthy activities that are too mild to be classified as effective aerobic exercise.

KEY TERMS

Adenosine Triphosphate	Exercise Training
Adherence	Fast-twitch Muscle Fibers
Aerobic	Glycogen
Aerobic Training	Lactate Threshold
Anaerobic	Lactic Acid
Blood Glucose	Maintenance Training
Cardiovascular Fitness	Podiatrist
Catecholamines	Recovery Energy Use
Circuit Resistance Training	Slow-twitch Muscle Fibers
Cool-down Period	Target Heart Rate
Dehydration	Ventilatory Threshold
Detraining	Warm-up Period

EXPLORING YOUR ACCESS TO HEALTH

" Fitness Scorecard "

Running is a popular physical activity, and the following inventory uses running to assess fitness. It is also appropriate to use other aerobic activities in place of running for this test. Circle the number of the statement under each category which best describes you.

CARDIOVASCULAR HEALTH*
Under medical care for heart or circulatory problems.	0
Such problems exist but medical care not required.	1
Past cardiovascular ailments have been pronounced "cured."	2
No history of cardiovascular trouble.	3

INJURIES**
Unable to do any strenuous work because of injury.	0
Level of activity is limited by the injury.	1
Some pain during activity but performance isn't affected significantly.	2
No injuries.	3

FIRST (OR MOST RECENT) RUN**
Able to run less than a half-mile or five minutes without stopping.	0
Ran between a half-mile and a mile (5 to 10 minutes) non-stop.	0
Completed between a mile and 1 1/2 miles (10 to 15 minutes) .	0

RUNNING BACKGROUND
Have never trained formally for running.	0
No running training within the last three years or more.	1
No running training within the last one to two years.	2
Have trained for running within the last year.	3

OTHER RELATED ACTIVITIES

    Not currently active in any regular sports or exercise programs.   0

    Regularly participate in "slow sports" such as golf, baseball, softball.   1

    Regularly practice vigorous "stop-and-go" sports such as tennis, basketball, soccer.   2

    Regularly participate in steady-paced, prolonged activities such as bicycling, hiking, swimming.   3

AGE

    50s and older.   0
    40s   1
    30s   2
    20s   3

WEIGHT

    More than 25 pounds above your "ideal" weight.   0
    16 to 25 pounds above your "ideal" weight.   1
    6 to 15 pounds of "ideal" weight.   2
    Within 5 pounds of "ideal" weight (or below ideal weight).   3

RESTING PULSE RATE

    80 beats per minute or higher   0
    In the 70s.   1
    In the 60s.   0
    In the 50s.   3

SMOKING

    A regular smoker.   0
    An occasional smoker.   1
    Have been a regular smoker but quit.   2
    Never have smoked regularly.   3

Total Score   _____

Exceptions

* If you have any history of heart or circulatory disease, do not continue with this series; participate in closely supervised activities.

** If these injuries or illnesses are temporary, wait until they are cured before starting the exercise program applicable to you. If they are chronic, adjust the program to fit your limitations.

*** If you can run continuously for 1 1/2 miles (15 minutes) or more, you may start a running or other exercise program at an intensity appropriate for you, no matter what you score is; you are fit!

Scoring

Total the number you circled and go the "Fitness Assessment" exercise in the next section for interpretation and application of your score.

Source: Adapted from *Runner's World,* January 19-3, 27. Used with permission.

ASSESSING HEALTH

1. **Fitness Assessment.** Note your total score on the "Fitness Scorecard." A score of 20 or higher is excellent. You probably can skip the preliminaries and go directly to a running (or other aerobic exercise) program. A score of 1() to 19 is average for adults. Start at the jogging or moderate exercise level. If you scored less than 10 points, you should forget about running and even jogging for now and concentrate on raising your score by walking or easing into exercise. Before beginning any exercise program, be sure to consult with your physician.

2. **Personal Fitness Plan.** Review the principles to consider in planning a cardiovascular fitness program discussed in your textbook. Plan and implement a (or modify your current) fitness program with clearly stated objectives, activities, and approaches to evaluating your progress. The self-assessment inventories in the preceding exercise provide a beginning point for planning and evaluating personal progress. Also, see Chapter 1 to assist you in planning for self-directed behavior.

3. **Activity Record.** Keep a written record of your physical activity for one month. Evaluate your activity in terms of the following elements of conditioning: warm-up, training level, fatigue, cooling down, and recovery. Periodically review your progress.

REVIEW TEST

Short Answer

1. List at least five benefits of aerobic exercise.

2. Differentiate between anaerobic and aerobic exercise.

3. List and briefly describe three physiological and three psychological benefits of aerobic exercise.

4. Discuss the points to keep in mind for adhering to an exercise program.

5. Offer five tips for initiating an exercise program.

6. Briefly describe how to calculate the target heart rate for exercising to improve aerobic capacity.

7. Differentiate between "fast-twitch" muscle fibers and "slow-twitch" muscle fibers.

8. Describe what is meant by "lactate threshold".

9. List two ways to determine exercise intensity.

10. Briefly discuss the dangers of exercising in hot and cold weather.

Fill-in-the-Blank

1. Carbohydrate in the blood is called _____ _____.

2. _____ _____ results when the intensity or pace of exercise causes a significant lactic acid accumulation in the blood.

3. The process in which the benefits of exercise begin to reverse and decline due to withdrawal from training is called _____.

4. Hormones that are released during exercise that have an inhibitory effect on appetite and arousal are called _____.

5. Large amounts of water loss during exercise in hot weather can lead to _____.

Multiple Choice

1. The optimal duration of an exercise session is:
   a. 15-20 minutes
   b. 20-25 minutes
   c. 30-45 minutes
   d. 45 -60 minutes

2. Which of the following is not a danger of exercising in cold weather?
   a. Angina pectoris
   b. Irregular heart beats
   c. Dehydration
   d. Expiratory strain

3. High intensity, short-burst activities in which the muscles rely heavily on the production of energy without adequate oxygen are called:
   a. Aerobic activities
   b. Cardiovascular fitness activities
   c. Anaerobic activities
   d. Endurance activities

4. The ability of the heart, lungs, and blood vessels to function efficiently can be improved by:
   a. Aerobic exercise
   b. Anaerobic exercise
   c. Flexibility
   d. Body Building

5. Activities which are low enough intensity so that they can be prolonged and use large amounts of oxygen are called:
   a. Anaerobic activities
   b. Aerobic activities
   c. Endurance activities
   d. Maintenance activities

6. Which of the following is not a physiological benefit of exercise?
   a. Improved heart function
   b. Increased longevity
   c. Increased metabolic rate
   d. Increased blood pressure

7. People who exercise regularly frequently report:
   a. Increased productivity
   b. An increased self-concept
   c. Relief from tension
   d. All of the above

8. Muscle fibers that produce large amounts of anaerobic energy but fatigue relative quickly are called:
   a. Slow-twitch muscle fibers
   b. Fast-twitch muscle fibers
   c. Aerobic muscle fibers
   d. Anaerobic muscle fibers

9. Exercise heart rate can be monitored by:
   a. Counting the pulses at the radial artery
   b. Counting the heart beats with the hand over the heart
   c. Using the RPE (rate of perceived exertion) scale
   d. All of the above

10. The most important piece of clothing for exercisers is:
    a. Footwear
    b. Free weights
    c. Rubberized sweatsuits
    d. Cotton clothing

CHAPTER 9

MUSCULAR FITNESS

CHAPTER OVERVIEW

Images of lean, muscular men and women have become very prevalent in the media. Memberships in health clubs have soared. Most people consider muscular strength and fitness to be a part of total fitness. While aerobic fitness is important, we must meet and maintain certain minimum standards of muscular strength for total fitness. Chapter 9 explores the types of muscular contractions that are essential to understanding the use of exercises to strengthen specific muscles. Improvement of muscular fitness generally requires the use of a greater overload resistance to stimulate the muscle to produce greater force. Chapter 9 discusses the methods of providing resistance, including static, isotonic, variable, isokinetic, and body weight. In addition, the principles and specific strategies are discussed for resistance training programs. Chapter 9 concludes with the utilization of games and sports competition to maintaining an active lifestyle.

LEARNING OBJECTIVES

Upon completion of Chapter 9 you should be able to:

1. List and describe the two basic types of muscular contractions.
2. Compare the advantages and disadvantages of each of the following types of muscular activity that provide overload resistance: static, isotonic, variable, isokinetic, and body weight.
3. Define the term "repetition" and discuss it's importance in resistance training.
4. Describe use of resistance for muscular strength development and the four phases of strength training.
5. Discuss how "power training" and "power resistance training" can be incorporated into a strength training regimen.
6. Describe muscular endurance training.
7. Discuss the importance of muscular balance, including testing and exercise programs to improve balance.
8. Describe the two processes required for muscle toning.
9. Discuss the use of resistance training to improve cardiovascular fitness.
10. Discuss circuit resistance training and the exercises for a total routine.
11. Describe the benefits and potential dangers of games and sports for improved performance and general fitness.

KEY TERMS

Concentric	Power Resistance Training
Constant Resistance	Power Training
Eccentric	Repetition
Isokinetic	Set
Isokinetic Resistance	Spot Reducing
Isotonic Resistance	Static Resistance
Muscular Balance	Strength Training
Muscular Endurance Training	Supercompensation
Periodization	Variable Resistance

EXPLORING YOUR ACCESS TO HEALTH

"Strength Training Log"

Muscular resistance training is beneficial for improving muscle strength. Keep a record of your strength training routine for a week:

Resistance Exercise(s)	Workload Level	Number of Repetitions	Number of Sets

Day 1:

Day 2:

Day 3:

Day 4:

Day 5:

Day 6:

Day 7:

ASSESSING HEALTH

1. **Strength Training Log.** As discussed in your textbook, everyday movements such as opening a stuck door or lifting a heavy box require a degree of muscular strength. While aerobic exercises are beneficial for improving the function of muscle groups used in the exercise, other muscles are generally not affected. Recreational games and sports can make fitness more enjoyable. Review your strength training log and identify areas that need improvement. Which specific resistance exercises would help to improve your particular game or sport?

2. **Personal Muscle Fitness Plan.** Review the principles to consider in planning a muscular fitness program discussed in your textbook. Plan and implement a (or modify your current) muscular fitness program with clearly stated objectives, activities, and approaches to evaluating your progress. Also, see Chapter 1 to assist you in planning for self-directed behavior.

3. **Muscle Fitness Assessment.** Arrange to have your muscular fitness assessed by an exercise specialist, such as an Exercise Physiologist, Physical Therapist, etc. Based on your results, plan a strength training program to improve your muscular fitness.

4. **Resource Guide.** Prepare a list of muscular fitness resources in your community. Possibly investigate you campus wellness program, public and private facilities, fitness assessment services, and places to purchase fitness equipment. Summarize your impressions of each resource.

REVIEW TEST

Short Answer

1. List the two basic types of muscular contractions.

2. Discuss the disadvantages of static resistance for muscular strength development.

3. Describe the role of games and sports for general fitness.

4. List at least two advantages and two disadvantages of isokinetic resistance training.

5. List three examples of body weight exercises.

6. Define "repetition" and describe the general principles of resistance training.

7. Describe how power training and power resistance training can be incorporated into a strength training program.

8. Discuss the importance of muscular balance in preventing muscular injury.

9. Describe the use of circuit resistance training for general and cardiovascular fitness.

10. Briefly describe circuit resistance training routine that is most beneficial for improving fitness.

Fill-in-the-Blank

1. Dynamic contractions in which the internal muscular tension is greater than the external resistance is called _____.

2. A _____ moving the resistance through one complete range of motion and returning to the starting position.

3. The use of strength exercises to tone a specific area of the body is called _____ _____.

4. _____ is mobilized from at least three areas in order of importance: Stomach (abdomen), Seat (gluteal), and Thigh (femoral).

5. Resistance that is immovable by the muscular force is termed _____ or _____.

87

Multiple Choice

1. Dynamic contractions in which the internal muscular tension is greater than the external resistance is called:
   a. Eccentric contractions
   b. Isotonic contractions
   c. Concentric contractions
   d. Endurance contractions

2. The dynamic contraction in which the muscle moves at a specific controlled speed is called:
   a. Isokinetic
   b. Isotonic
   c. Eccentric
   d. Concentric

3. Which of the following is not a body weight bearing exercise?
   a. Sit-up
   b. Push-up
   c. Lifting a barbell free-weight
   d. Running

4. The best type of resistance exercise system for producing a desirable aerobic effect is:
   a. Circuit resistance training
   b. Body weight bearing exercises
   c. Muscular endurance training
   d. Power training

5. The type of resistance that provides the muscle with stress only at a specific point in the range of motion is called:
   a. Dynamic
   b. Static
   c. Concentric
   d. Eccentric

6. The use of standard free-weight barbells and dumbbells are examples of:
   a. Isometric resistance
   b. Isokinetic resistance
   c. Isotonic resistance
   d. Static resistance

7. The use of resistance that is altered throughout the range of motion in an attempt to match the changing capabilities of muscle at different joint angles is called:
   a. Static resistance
   b. Muscular function resistance
   c. Variable resistance
   d. Isometric resistance

8. The total circuit resistance training conditioning program is _____ times per week.
   a. 1
   b. 3
   c. 5
   d. 7

9. The type of resistance that provides a "constant load" on the muscle throughout the entire range of motion is called:
   a. Isometric
   b. Isokinetic
   c. Isotonic
   d. Dynamic

10. Which of the following can add an additional negative load on the heart during activity?
    a. A plastic sweating suit
    b. Jogging after loose balls in tennis
    c. Jogging up and down a basketball court
    d. All of the above

CHAPTER 10

ADDICTIONS AND ADDICTIVE BEHAVIOR

CHAPTER OVERVIEW

Though once limited only to drugs, the most commonly recognized addictions today involve the use of alcohol or other drugs, food, sex, relationships, gambling, spending, and work. Addiction may develop when a behavior produces a positive mood change, no matter how minor. Chapter 10 explores the addictive process which involves four major features: 1) involvement, 2) loss of control, 3) denial, and 4) relapse. While numerous theories have attempted to identify a single factor, there are no single factors that produce the disease of addiction. Chapter 10 discusses the theories of addiction from biological and psychosocial models. The effects of any addictive behavior are not limited to the individual addict. On the contrary, the families and society are also exposed to the harmful consequences of this disease. Individuals who are from addictive families have an increased risk of developing their own addiction. Often, the families become codependent and enable an addict to maintain their addictive behavior. Finally, Chapter 10 discusses the interventions that are used in the treatment of addictive behaviors, including inpatient or outpatient care, individual and group therapy, and self-help treatments such as the 12-step programs.

LEARNING OBJECTIVES

Upon completion of Chapter 10 you should be able to:

1. Define "addiction" and the three criteria for diagnosing addiction.
2. Briefly describe the four major features of addiction.
3. Discribe the five progressive stages of addiction.
4. Discuss the characteristics of individuals most likely to become addicted to alcohol.
5. Define tolerance.
6. Describe at least three behavioral compulsive behaviors.
7. Discuss the two categories of theories concerning the cause of addiction.
8. Describe the effects of addiction in the family and society.
9. Define Post Traumatic Shock Disorder and list four symptoms of this disorder.
10. Define the term "codependency" and its relationship to dysfunctional family systems.
11. Describe the purpose of intervention and strategies to intervene in an addict's denial system.
12. List the components of successful treatment programs.
12. Discuss the twelve steps of addiction recovery programs.

KEY TERMS

Addiction	Post-traumatic Stress Disorder
Codependency	Social Learning Theory
Denial	Tolerance
Enabler	Withdrawal

EXPLORING YOUR ACCESS TO HEALTH

"Do You Have a Chemical Dependency Problem?

Check all of the following responses that apply to you:

1. I look forward to getting together with my friends to drink or use drugs. _____
2. I look forward to holidays and other social occasions because it's a time to drink or use drugs. _____
3. I am drinking alcohol or using drugs more often than I have in the past. _____
4. I am drinking more alcohol or using more drugs to achieve the same effects than I have in the past. _____
5. Alcohol or drugs are frequently used with I am with my friends and/or family. _____
6. I have had at least one time with I do not remember things that have happened during a drinking or drug using episode. _____
7. Some of the significant people in my life (i.e., friends, family, employers, etc.) have told me that they are concerned about my drinking or drug use. _____
8. Most of my friends are heavy users of alcohol or drugs. _____
9. I think that I might have a problem handling my alcohol or drug use. _____
10. I only go to restaurants that serve alcohol. _____
11. I have driven a car while intoxicated or under the influence of alcohol or drugs but have never been arrested. _____
12. I have been arrested for driving a car while intoxicated or under the influence of alcohol or drugs. _____
13. At times I have had problems paying my bills because I have spent my money on alcohol or alcohol. _____
14. I feel guilty when I drink alcohol or use drugs. _____
15. Sometimes I do things while I have been drinking or using drugs that I later regret. _____
16. I have lied to the significant people in my life about my alcohol or drug use. _____
17. Sometimes I do not remember what I have done while I have used alcohol or drugs. _____
18. I prefer to drink or use drugs when I am alone. _____
19. There are times that I have to lie or conceal my alcohol or drug use. _____
20. I have missed work because of my drinking or drug use. _____

Scoring

Note the statements that you checked and go to the "Do You Have a Chemical Dependency Problem?" in the next section for the interpretation.

ASSESSING HEALTH

1. **"Do You Have a Chemical Dependency Problem?"** The use of alcohol and drugs is so common place in our society that most people do not realize when they may have developed a chemical dependency problem. If you checked any three of the statements, you may have a chemical dependency problem. If you checked any five, then you have a greater likelihood of having a chemical dependency problem. If you have checked seven or more there is a strong likelihood that you may have a problem with chemical dependency and should seek professional help.

2. **How to Tell Whether Someone You Know is Chemically Dependent.** The questionnaire you completed in the previous section is comprised of personality traits which researchers have found in common among people with addictions. Such addictions are not limited to drugs, but could include a variety of substances or behaviors. If you anwered "Yes" to a few or many of the items, it does not necessarily mean that you will develop an addiction. Most people do not become addicts. Rather, consider those traits you have in common with addicted persons and how you could modify your behavior or view of yourself in positive ways. If you do have an addiction to such things as food, tobacco, alcohol, drugs, or other behaviors, consider how making changes could help in kicking the habit. Write these potential changes as behavioral goals and perhaps focus upon one or more for a self-change project (see Chapter 1 of this workbook).

2. **Looking Further.** Select and abstract a journal article from the library which reports research or discusses some aspect of addictive behavior (i.e., substance abuse, alcoholic abuse, eating disorders, etc.). The abstract should include the purpose of the article/study, the research methods used or major concepts presented, the results and/or conclusions arrived at by the author, and your remarks about the implications of the information for your personal health.

REVIEW TEST

Short Answer

1. Define "addiction" and list the three criteria for a diagnosis of an addiction.

2. Describe the five progressive stages of addiction.

3. List the four major features of addiction.

4. Briefly describe what is meant in the addictive relationship as "nurturing through avoidance."

5. Briefly discuss the two categories of theories concerning the cause of addictive behavior.

6. Describe how co-dependency and enabling contribute to an addict's behaviors.

7. Define "tolerance."

8. Describe at least three behavioral compulsive behaviors.

9. Briefly describe the effects of addiction on the family.

10. Describe the purpose of intervention and strategies to intervene in an addict's denial system.

Fill-in-the-Blank

1. Initially, _____ _____ provide a sense of pleasure or stability that is beyond the control of the addict.

2. In order to be addictive, a behavior must have the potential to produce a _____ _____ _____.

3. The four major features of addiction are:

    a) _____, b) _____,

    c) _____, and d) _____.

4. _____ is the most serious addiction.

5. The inability to see the truth is called _____.

Multiple Choice

1. A series of temporary physical and psychological symptoms that occur when the addict stops the addictive behavior is known as:
    a. Physiological dependence
    b. Withdrawal
    c. Tolerance
    d. Addiction

2. Dependence on a substance or behavior to produce a desired mood and manage emotions is called a(n):
   a. Addiction
   b. Withdrawal
   c. Abstinence Syndrome
   d. Tolerance

3. The most serious addiction is:
   a. Gambling
   b. Alcohol
   c. Cocaine
   d. Tobacco

4. A condition experienced by people who have been subjected to levels of trauma beyond the range of normal is called:
   a. Obsessive/compulsive disorder
   b. Abstinence disorder
   c. Post-traumatic stress disorder
   d. Hypervigilance

5. The phenomenon in which progressively larger doses of a drug are needed to produce the desired effects is called:
   a. Tolerance
   b. Withdrawal
   c. Dependency
   d. Addiction

6. The model of addiction that proposes that people learn addictive behaviors by watching parents, caregivers, and significant others is known as:
   a. Societal Influences model
   b. Stimulus-Response model
   c. Social Learning model
   d. Behavioral Intent model

7. The relationship pattern in which a person is thought to be "addicted to the addict" is known as:
   a. Enabling
   b. Codependent
   c. Post-traumatic stress
   d. Control-Controller relationship

8. A person who knowingly or unknowingly protects addicts from the natural consequences of their behavior are:
   a. Enablers
   b. Addicts
   c. Dependents
   d. Codependents

9. The most effective treatment for addictions is:
   a. Individual counseling
   b. Group and family therapy
   c. Education
   d. All of the above

10. Which of the following is not a step in the twelve steps of addiction recovery programs?
    a. We are powerless over [alcohol], and that our lives have been unmanageable.
    b. We came to believe that a power greater than ourselves can restore use to sanity.
    c. We can rely on nobody to help us overcome our addiction.
    d. We humbly ask God to remove our shortcomings.

CHAPTER 11

ALCOHOL AND TOBACCO

CHAPTER OVERVIEW

Alcohol is the most widely used and abused recreational drug in our society. Used by approximately 70% of all Americans, this drug can impair judgment and coordination. Furthermore, emotional and intellectual functioning may be impaired with the use of alcohol. While most of us recognize the potential harmful effects of alcohol consumption, we deny that such problems can happen to us. Similarly, our society legally sanctions the liberal use of certain substances such as tobacco. Smoking is the most common form of tobacco use and delivers a strong dose of nicotine to the user, along with an additional 4,000 chemical substances. Chapter 11 investigates alcohol as a drug, how it is manufactured and metabolized, as well as the immediate and long-term effects of alcohol abuse. In addition, Chapter 11 explores the disease of alcoholism, the costs of this disease to both the individual and society, and the current intervention strategies. In addition, Chapter 11 examines the health hazards of smoking and the benefits of quitting.

LEARNING OBJECTIVES

Upon completion of Chapter 11 you should be able to:

1. Discuss alcohol use and its associated problems in our society.
2. Describe alcohol in terms of its chemical name, production, and forms in which it is consumed.
3. Discuss the metabolization process of alcohol by the body.
4. Briefly describe the guidelines for communicating concern about alcohol abuse when someone close to you drinks too much.
5. Discuss the factors that can affect BAC and tests used to determine its level in the body.
6. Describe the physiological and psychological effects of alcohol.
7. Describe the effects of alcohol on pregnancy.
8. Discuss the causes and characteristics of alcoholism and its consequent problems.
9. Discuss the effects of alcoholism on the family.
10. List the various reasons why alcoholics seek help.
11. Discuss the treatment of alcoholism focusing on the family's role, treatment programs and facilities, and drug therapy.
12. Describe "nicotine," its physiological effects, and the products in which it is consumed.
13. Describe the constituents of tobacco smoke and its physiological effects.
14. Discuss the effects of smoking on such diseases as cancer and heart disease.

15. Discuss the hazards of "secondhand smoke" and the steps to protect against "passive smoking."
16. Describe how the forms of tobacco consumption and the associated health risks are changing in our society.
17. Describe "nicotine withdrawal" and how nicotine gum acts to assist the quitter.
18. Discuss the social issues surrounding tobacco production and marketing.

KEY TERMS

Alcohol Abuse (Alcoholism)
Alcoholics Anonymous
Blood Alcohol Concentration (BAC)
Binge Drinking
Blackout
Carbon Monoxide
Chewing Tobacco
Delirium Tremens (DT)
Distillation
Emphysema
Ethyl Alcohol (Ethanol)
Fermentation
Hangover

Intervention
Learned Behavioral Tolerance
Leukoplakia
Nicotine
Nicotine Poisoning
Nicotine Withdrawal
Peripheral Vascular Disease
Platelet Adhesiveness
Proof
Secondhand Smoke
Snuff
Sudden Infant Death Syndrome
Tar

EXPLORING YOUR ACCESS TO HEALTH

"Responsible Drinking Behaviors"

If you drink alcoholic beverages at least occasionally, assess how responsibly you drink by answering "Yes" or "No" to the following questions.

1. Have you mixed alcoholic beverages with other drugs? _____

2. Have you used alcoholic beverages to relieve depression? _____

3. Do you ever drink alcoholic beverages rapidly? _____

4. Do you drink alcoholic beverages without food? _____

5. Have you ever driven after drinking? _____

6. Have you ever turned to alcoholic beverages to relax? _____

7. Have you ever consumed alcohol to the point of vomiting, passing out, or not remembering what you did while drinking? _____

8. Have you served alcohol to others who were already intoxicated? _____

9. Do you ever encourage or push others to drink? _____

10. Have you ever sponsored a "kegger," "beer blast," or other social function centered around drinking? _____

11. Have you ever ridden with an intoxicated driver? _____

12. Do you ever play "drinking games"? _____

13. Have you ever gotten into a fight, acted obnoxiously or obscenely, or engaged in vandalism while drinking? _____

14. Do you ever drink because someone else pushes or encourages you? _____

Scoring

Note the questions to which you answered "Yes" and turn to the "Responsible Drinking" exercise in the next section.

"Your Attitudes Toward Tobacco Use"

If you use tobacco in any form, complete the following test by circling the number that corresponds to how you feel about each statement. Smoking, chewing, etc., may be substituted for the words "tobacco use."

	Strongly Agree	Mildly Agree	Mildly Disagree	Strongly Disagree
1. Tobacco use is not nearly as dangerous as many other health hazards.	1	2	3	4
2. I don't use tobacco enough to get any of the diseases that cigarette smoking is supposed to cause.	1	2	3	4
3. If a person has already used tobacco for many years, it probably won't do much good to stop.	1	2	3	4
4. It would be hard for me to give up tobacco use.	1	2	3	4
5. Tobacco use is enough of a health hazard for something to be done about it.	4	3	2	1
6. The kind of tobacco I use is much less likely than other kinds to give me any of the diseases that tobacco is supposed to cause.	1	2	3	4

7. As soon as a person quits using tobacco he or she begins to recover from much of the damage that smoking has caused.	4	3	2	1
8. It would be hard for me to cut down to half the amount of tobacco I now use.	4	3	2	1
9. The whole problem of tobacco use and health is a very minor one.	1	2	3	4
10. I haven't used tobacco long enough to worry about the diseases that tobacco use is supposed to cause.	1	2	3	4
11. Quitting tobacco use helps a person to live longer.	4	3	2	1
12. It would be difficult for me to make any substantial change in my tobacco use habits.	1	2	3	4

Scoring

Write the number you circled after each statement in the space below. Then total the scores for each column. Turn to the "Attitudes Toward Tobacco" exercise in the next section for interpretation of your score.

Importance	Personal Relevance	Value of Stopping	Capability of Stopping
1) ____	2) ____	3) ____	4) ____
5) ____	6) ____	7) ____	8) ____
9) ____	10) ____	11) ____	12) ____

Source: Adapted from "Testing Your Attitudes Toward Smoking" (National Clearinghouse for Smoking and Health).

ASSESSING HEALTH

1. **Responsible Drinking.** Review your answers on the "Responsible Drinking Behaviors" questionnaire. The questions reflect irresponsible drinking behaviors and, therefore, you should give special attention to the items to which you answered "Yes." Consider how you will drink more responsibly in the future. General guidelines for responsible drinking include:

a. Drinking along with other activities and not using alcohol for its own sake.

b. Avoiding intoxication by drinking slowly, with food in your stomach, and carefully monitoring your reactions.

c. Acknowledging another's right to choose whether or not to drink. Never push drinks and also serve alternative non-alcoholic beverages.

d. Avoiding the use of alcohol in combination with other drugs.

e. Never driving after drinking. Always have a "designated driver" or other transportation available.

f. Seeking help if you think you may have a drinking problem and encouraging others to seek help if you suspect they may have a problem.

2. **Attitudes Toward Tobacco Use.** Refer to your scores on the "Your Attitudes Toward Tobacco Use" inventory. Your scores correspond to the four factors typically involved in quitting the tobacco habit: importance, personal relevance, value of stopping, and capability of stopping. A score of 9 or more for any of the factors indicates that your attitude about the factor will be important in a successful effort to stop using tobacco. Scores of 6 or less indicate that the factor is not important to your quitting. Go back to the individual items in each of the categories to which you scored 9 or above and assess how you might change your attitudes to facilitate quitting.

3. **Self-Change Plan.** Self-knowledge about alcohol, and/or tobacco consumption can set the stage for modifying your intake of these substances. If appropriate, you may want to select one of these chemical dependencies as the focus for a health behavior change project. Your textbook discusses approaches and resources to assist you in the process, and Chapter 1 of this workbook provides a systematic format for self-behavior change.

REVIEW TEST

Short Answer

1. Give examples of the various forms of tobacco consumption and their associated health risks.

2. Describe "nicotine" and its physiological effects.

3. Discuss alcohol and its associated problems in our society.

4. Discuss alcohol in terms of its chemical name, production, and forms in which it is consumed.

5. Describe the metabolism process of alcohol by the body.

6. List several problems of nonsmokers which are directly associated with secondhand smoke.

7. Describe "nicotine withdrawal" and how nicotine gum acts to assist the quitter.

8. Describe the causes and characteristics of alcoholism and consequent problems.

9. Discuss the social issues surrounding tobacco production and marketing.

10. Discuss the treatment of alcoholism, focusing on the family's role, treatment programs and facilities, and drug therapy.

Fill-in-the-Blank

1. Ethanol may be produced by the process of _____ in which plant sugars are broken down by yeast organisms.

2. Alcohol is metabolized by the _____ (organ).

3. _____ _____ _____ babies suffer from mental retardation, small head size, and other birth defects.

4. Cigarette smoke is composed of 92% _____ which displaces the oxygen-carrying capacity of red blood cells.

5. _____ is the thick, brownish substance that is condensed from particulate matter in cigarette smoke.

Multiple Choice

1. The most widely used and abused drug in our society is:
   a. Nicotine
   b. Caffeine
   c. Alcohol
   d. Amphetamines

2. The active chemical in alcohol is:
   a. Ethyl alcohol
   b. Isopropyl alcohol
   c. Ether
   d. Distilled spirits

3. A colorless liquid that turns brown upon oxidation is:
   a. Tar
   b. Nicotine
   c. Chewing tobacco
   d. Quid

4. Most wines are:
   a. 14% - 16% alcohol
   b. 12% - 15% alcohol
   c. 8% - 10% alcohol
   d. 2% - 6% alcohol

5. The most common form of tobacco use is:
   a. Chewing tobacco
   b. Snuff
   c. Smoking
   d. All of the above

6. The majority of alcohol is absorbed into the blood stream in the:
   a. Mouth
   b. Stomach
   c. Small intestine
   d. Large intestine

7. A temporary form of amnesia usually occurring at higher levels of intoxication is called:
   a. Blackouts
   b. Hangovers
   c. Delirium tremens
   d. Binge drinking

8. The effect that nicotine has on the central nervous system is a:
   a. Stimulant
   b. Analgesic
   c. Depressant
   d. Hallucinogenic

9. A chronic disease in which the alveoli are destroyed, making breathing difficult is:
   a. Chronic Obstructive Lung Disorder
   b. Stroke
   c. Emphysema
   d. Sudden Infant Death Syndrome

10. A condition characterized by leatherly white patches inside the mouth produced by contact with the irritants in tobacco juice is known as:
    a. Leukoplakia
    b. Neoplasm
    c. Dental fissures
    d. Oral cancer

CHAPTER 12

PRESCRIPTION, OVER-THE-COUNTER AND ILLEGAL DRUGS

CHAPTER OVERVIEW

We live in the pharmaceutical age, where a "quick fix" is available for virtually every ache, pain, and uncomfortable mood that we may experience. As consumers, we must have an accurate knowledge in order to make informed judgments about drug use. Similarly, illicit drugs offer a convenient way to alter the consciousness to a "high," enhancing the pleasure of an activity or relieving an unpleasant mood. However, the use of illicit drugs can have physical, emotional, social, and legal consequences. Chapter 12 describes the six categories of drugs and their effect on the human body. Since thousands of prescription drugs are available for physicians to prescribe for patients, there may be a tendency for overmedicating or overprescribing drugs. Therefore, it is important that consumers work with their physicians to avoid complications associated with prescription medications. Over-the-counter drugs are readily available and there is increased risk of complications when these drugs are not used appropriately. Chapter 12 further discusses the effects of various illicit drugs currently used in America, their physical and psychological effects, and the issues related to drug usage.

LEARNING OBJECTIVES

Upon completion of Chapter 12 you should be able to:

1. Describe the currently accepted explanation of drug action.
2. List, describe, and give examples of each of the six drug categories.
3. Differentiate between drug "use" and "abuse."
4. List the four most hazardous drug interactions.
5. List the major routes of drug administration.
6. List, describe, and give examples of the classifications of prescription drugs commonly of interest to college students.
7. Discuss the use of generic drugs and the advantages these alternative medications provide consumers.
8. Discuss OTC drugs in terms of popularity, safety, efficacy, and labeling.
9. List the general precautions for OTC users.
10. Give a general overview of illicit drug use.
11. List several reasons why people use illicit drugs.
12. List the five representative categories of illicit drugs and give at least two examples of drugs in each category.
13. Describe cocaine, crack, freebase, crank, and ice in terms of their use, physical and psychological effects, and social costs.

14. Describe marijuana, its popularity, various forms, and physical and psychological effects.
15. Describe the history of opiate use, its physical and psychological effects, and treatment for addiction.
16. Discuss the use of psychedelics, the forms in which they are consumed, and their physical and psychological effects.
17. List and describe the deliriants and their physical and psychological effects.
18. List and describe Designer Drugs.
19. Describe the use of inhalants and solvents, the forms in which they are used, and the associated dangers.
20. Describe the scope of the illicit drug problem in the United States.
21. List and describe the possible solutions to the illicit drug problem.

KEY TERMS

Amphetamines
Amyl Nitrite
Analgesics
Anaphylactic Shock
Antagonism
Antibiotics
Antidepressants
Black Tar Heroin
Caffeine
Caffeinism
CNS Depressant
Cocaine
Codeine
Commercial Preparations
Crack
Crank
Cross-Tolerance
Deliriant
Delirium
Designer Drug
Diuretic
Drug
Drug Abuse
Drug Misuse
Endorphins
Freebase
Generic Drugs
Ghanja
Hallucination
Hashish
Herbal Preparations
Heroin
Ice
Illicit Drugs

Injection
Intolerance
Intramuscular Injection
Intravenous Injection
Inunction
Laxative
Lysergic Acid Diethylamide (LSD)
Marijuana
Mescaline
Methadone Maintenance
Morphine
Narcotics
Opium
Oral Ingestion
Over-The-Counter (OTC) Drugs
Peyote
Phencyclidine (PCP)
Polydrug Use
Prescription Drugs
Prostaglandin Inhibitors
Psilocybin
Psychedelics
Psychoactive Drugs
Rebound Effect
Receptor Sites
Reticular Formation
Route of Administration
Sedatives
Set
Setting
Subcutaneous Injection
Suppositories
Synesthesia
Tetrahydrocannabinol (THC)

Inhalation   Tranquilizers
Inhalants and Solvents   Xanthines
Inhibition

EXPLORING YOUR ACCESS TO HEALTH

"Product Information Record"

Obtain a copy of the current *Physician's Desk Reference* from a library or local bookstore. Read the product information for the generic or brand-name medications which you or a family member are presently taking or have taken in the recent past. Product information inserts are also available from your pharmacist. A medical dictionary may be helpful for interpreting this information. List and describe each product on the following form.

Brand Name	Generic Name	Indications	Contra-Indicators	Side Effects

Scoring

For interpretation and application of the information you recorded above, turn to the exercise entitled "Physician's Desk Reference" in the next section.

"Illicit Drug Assessment"

For each of the following illicit drugs, note the route of administration, effects, and physical and psychological dependence.

Drug	Route of Administration	Effects	Dependence
Cocaine			
Freebase			
Crack			
Crank			
Ice			
Marijuana			
Heroin			
LSD			
Mescaline			
MDMA			
Amyl Nitrite			

ASSESSING HEALTH

1. **Medication Pricing.** Research the prices of OTC and prescription drugs with which you are familiar. Compare the costs of the brand-name products with store brand and generic preparations containing the same active ingredients. Ask a pharmacists about "dispense-as-written" laws in your state and whether or not the pharmacist would honor a consumer's request for a generic substitution without specific permission from the prescribing physician.

2. **Product Information Record.** Review your entries on the "Product Information Record." Give particular attention to the contraindications and potential side effects. Consider the value of this information for consumers and whether or not your physician and pharmacist typically provide these data. Are there generic substitutions for any of the brand-name drugs? Are there potential adverse interactions between any of the products if used simultaneously?

3. **Illicit Drug Assessment.** Review the drugs in the "Illicit Drug Assessment." Consider the implications of drug use in the workplace. How might the use of illicit drugs affect the performance and safety of the user and others who might be involved indirectly? What about professions that involve the public safety (i.e., school bus drivers, airplane pilots, train engineers, etc.)? Should there be mandatory drug testing of all individuals to ensure safety?

4. **Recognizing Drug-Abuse Tendencies.** Complete the "Recognizing Drug-Abuse Tendencies" in your textbook. Consider your responses to each question and list a nondrug alternative to your feelings.

REVIEW TEST

Short Answer

1. Describe the currently accepted explanation of drug action.

2. List and describe the six categories of drugs.

3. Describe the damaging effects of cocaine use.

4. Briefly discuss the controversy surrounding methadone maintenance programs.

5. Discuss the use of generic drugs and the advantages these alternative medications provide consumers.

6. List the five representative categories of illicit drugs.

7. List and describe the commonly used classifications of OTC preparations.

8. List the three major reasons why people use illicit drugs.

9. Describe cocaine, crack, freebase, crank, and ice and discuss their use, physical and psychological effects, and social costs.

10. List alternatives to drugs for the purpose of pain relief.

Fill-in-the-Blank

1. A coffee drinker who experiences chronic insomnia, jitters, irritability, nervousness, anxiety, and/or involuntary muscle twitches is likely suffering from _____.

2. _____ occurs when drugs combine in the body to produce extremely uncomfortable reactions.

3. The small, hard chip of cocaine is called _____.

4. Psilocybin is the active chemical derived from the "magic _____."

5. Drugs which increase the excretion of urine from the body are called _____.

Multiple Choice

1. Drugs that can be purchased in pharmacies, supermarkets, or discount stores without a physician's prescription are called:
    a. Commercial drugs
    b. Recreational drugs
    c. Herbal drugs
    d. Over-the-counter drugs

2. Which of the following is a side effect of the xanthines:
    a. Increased appetite
    b. Decreased oxygen consumption
    c. Dizziness
    d. Decreased heart muscle contractions

3. Drugs that relieve pain are called:
    a. Depressants
    b. Stimulants
    c. Narcotics
    d. Psychedelics

4. The most frequently used route of administration of drugs is:
    a. Inhalation
    b. Oral
    c. Intravenous injection
    d. Subcutaneous injection

5. Opiatelike hormones that are manufactured in the human brain and contribute to feelings of well-being are:
   a. Endorphins
   b. Morphine
   c. Methadone
   d. Heroin

6. Drugs that are used to relieve pain are classified as:
   a. Analgesics
   b. Antibiotics
   c. Depressants
   d. Psychoactives

7. An example of a central nervous system depressant is:
   a. Morphine
   b. Acetaminophen
   c. Sedatives
   d. Amphetamines

8. Which of the following is a symptom of caffeinism?
   a. Irritability
   b. Headaches
   c. Involuntary muscle twitches
   d. All of the above

9. The active ingredient in OTC stimulants is:
   a. Amphetamines
   b. Caffeine
   c. Phenylpropanolamine
   d. Pyrilamine maleate

10. An image (auditory or visual) that is perceived but is not real is called a:
    a. Blackout
    b. Flashback
    c. Synesthesia
    d. Hallucination

CHAPTER 13

CARDIOVASCULAR DISEASE AND CANCER: UNDERSTANDING YOUR RISKS

CHAPTER OVERVIEW

Cardiovascular disease (CVD), cancer, and stroke are among the leading causes of death in the United States. Unlike communicable diseases, these chronic afflictions are to a great extent diseases of lifestyle. Some risk factors are unalterable and not under our control, such as our family history, age, sex, or race. Chapter 13 examines the alterable risk factors that are under our control that are a part of a health-promoting lifestyle. The factors for CVD and strokes include cigarette smoking, blood fat and cholesterol levels, hypertension, diet, exercise, obesity, diabetes, and emotional stress. Similarly, Chapter 13 describes the numerous factors that can lead to the development of cancer, including oncogenes, biological factors, occupational factors, social and psychological factors, diet, viruses, radiation, and combined risks. Taking action to alter our lifestyle can reduce our risk of CVD, cancers and strokes. Chapter 13 explores the most common types of heart diseases, their diagnosis, and current treatments. Furthermore, the various types of cancer and the current available treatments are examined.

LEARNING OBJECTIVES

Upon completion of Chapter 13 you should be able to:

1. Give an overview of the CVD problem.
2. Describe normal heart activity and trace the circulation of blood.
3. List the risk factors for CVD and describe their contribution to the disease process.
5. Describe a myocardial infarction, the possible immediate causes, and what can be done to assist the heart attack victim.
6. Discuss the following CVD's in terms of disease process, cause, and treatment: arrhythmias, angina pectoris, congestive heart failure, congenital heart disease, and stroke.
9. Discuss the advantages and disadvantages of angioplasty and bypass surgery.
10. Describe the process by which malignant and benign tumors develop and how cancer spreads through the system.
11. Describe the biological, occupational, social, psychological, and dietary factors which may contribute to the development of cancer.
12. List the American Cancer Society's nutritional guidelines for cancer prevention.
13. Discuss the carcinogenic potential of viruses, oncogenes, radiation, and combined risk factors.
14. Differentiate between the typical classifications of cancer.

15. Discuss the following types of cancer in terms of incidence, cause, treatment, and prevention: lung cancer, breast cancer, colon and rectal cancers, skin cancer, testicular cancer, pancreatic cancer, leukemia, and uterine cancer.
16. List the words of "Caution" in the seven warning signals of cancer.
17. Describe the available cancer treatment options.

KEY TERMS

Angina Pectoris	Heart Attack
Angiography	Hypertension
Angioplasty	Magnetic Resonance Imagery
Arrhythmia	Malignant
Arteries	Metastasis
Atria	Murmurs
Benign	Mutant Cells
Biopsy	Neoplasm
Cancer	Oncogenes
Capillaries	Oncologists
Carcinogens	Position Emissions Tomography (PET)
Cardiovascular Diseases	Radiotherapy
Cardiovascular System	Rheumatic Heart Disease
Chemotherapy	Stroke
Computerized Axial Tomography	Systolic Pressure
Congenital Heart Disease	Transient Ischemic Attacks
Coronary Bypass Surgery	Tumor
Coronary Thrombosis	Veins
Diastolic Pressure	Ventricles
Electrocardiogram (ECG)	Virulent
Embolus	Xeroradiograms
Epidemiologists	

EXPLORING YOUR ACCESS TO HEALTH

"Type-A Behavior Quiz"

Circle the number on the continuum that best characterizes your behavior for each item.

1. Casual about   1 2 3 4 5 6 7   Never late. appointments.

2. Not competitive 1 2 3 4 5 6 7   Very competitive.

3. Never feel   1 2 3 4 5 6 7   Always rushed even under pressure.

4.	Take things one at a time.	1	2	3	4	5	6	7	Try to do many things at once, think about what I'm going to do next.
5.	Slow doing things.	1	2	3	4	5	6	7	Fast (eating, walking, etc.)
6.	"Sit" on my feelings.	1	2	3	4	5	6	7	Express my feelings.
7.	Many interests outside school.	1	2	3	4	5	6	7	Few interests outside school.

Total (add the numbers you circled): _____

Score (multiply score by 3): _____

Scoring

For interpretation and application of your score, go to the exercise entitled "Type-A Behavior" in the next section.

Source: Adapted from Bortner, R. W. (1969). A short rating scale as a potential measure of pattern A behavior. *Journal of Chronic Disease*, 22, 87-91. Reprinted with permission.

"Warning Signals of Cancer"

Take some time to conduct a self-assessment of the following signs and symptoms for cancer. Indicate the presence or absence of any of these signals by responding "Yes" or "No."

1. Change in the size, texture, or color of a wart or mole. Persistent swelling, warmth, or redness of the skin. _____

2. A sore that does not heal or that heals slowly. _____

3. Unusual or unexplained bleeding or discharge from the bowel, nipples, or vagina or the presence of blood in the urine. _____

4. Thickening or lump in the breast, lip, tongue, testicle, or elsewhere. Changes in the skin or nipple of the breast. _____

5. Indigestion that persists, loss of appetite, unexplained weight loss, or unusual weakness. _____

6. Obvious change in bowel or bladder habits. Persistent diarrhea or constipation or bladder retention, incontinence, or frequent or painful urination. _____

7. Nagging or persistent cough, hoarseness, shortness of breath, difficulty swallowing, blood in sputum, or chest pain. _____

Scoring

For interpretation of your responses to this inventory, proceed to the exercise entitled, "Early Detection."

Source : Based upon recommendations for early detection of cancer, American Cancer Society.

ASSESSING HEALTH

1. **Type-A Behavior.** Although subject to continuing scientific debate about causative association, there is research which suggests that Type-A personalities have significantly greater representation among heart attack victims than persons with Type-B personalities. The Type-A personality has been described as aggressive, competitive, hostile, and lacking the ability to only focus on one task at a time. The Type-B personality is depicted by a behavior pattern which tends to be the opposite of Type-A.

   After completing the "Type-A Behavior Quiz," find your score and interpretation on the following key:

Score	Interpretation
More than 120	Very strongly Type-A
106 - 119	Definitely Type-A
100 - 105	Type-A, but the Type-B in you may save your life.
90 - 99	Type-B, but some Type-A tendencies.
Less than 90	Type-B

   If you scored in the Type-A range, what changes could you make to become more Type-B? Read about "hot reactors" and Type-A behavior in your textbook. Are you a hot or cold reactor? Notice that the suggested prevention techniques are applicable to both Type-A and hot reactor personalities.

2. **Cardiovascular Disease Prevention.** The risk factors for CVD are discussed in your textbook. Make a brief personal assessment for each of the following factors and summarize the change you can make to reduce your risks to CVD. For example, what are your risks regarding the unalterable risk factors? How will knowing this information assist you in CVD prevention?

Cigarette Smoking

Blood Fat Levels

Hypertension

Exercise

Diet and Obesity

Diabetes

Emotional Stress

Unalterable Risk Factors

3. **Early Detection.** A key factor in the early detection of cancer is periodic self-examination to evaluate any changes from normal. For example, conducting regular breast self-examination (females and males) and self-testicular examination (males) are musts (see your textbook). Of course, to detect such changes requires adequate "baseline" knowledge of what looks and feels "normal" for you.

   The American Cancer Society (ACS) has suggested seven warning signals of cancer (see your textbook). The signs and symptoms presented in the "Warning Signals of Cancer" in inventory are expanded versions of the ACS signals and provide a good basis for conducting self-examination and self-monitoring. Although these signals are not necessarily indications of cancer, if any one or more persist for several weeks, you should consult a physician. Also, the number or severity of the detected changes would dictate the immediacy of need for seeking medical assistance.

4. **Cancer Prevention.** The probable causes of cancer are discussed in your textbook. Below, make a brief personal assessment for each category and summarize the steps you can take to reduce your risks. For example, under "Biological Factors," describe your family history of cancer and how knowing this information can help you in cancer prevention.

Biological Factors

Occupational Factors

Social and Psychological Factors

Diet

Viral Causes

Oncogenes

Radiation

Combined Factors

5. **Looking Further.** Investigate the programs and services in your community that are directed at CVD (i.e., County Health Department, American Heart Association, American Red Cross Association, Paramed Foundation, etc.). Determine the goals and/or objectives of these programs and the services offered through their organization. Consider enrolling in a community Cardiopulmonary Resuscitation or First Aid course through your college/university or community organization.

REVIEW TEST

Short Answer

1. Briefly explain the CVD problem.

2. List the nine most common forms of CVD.

3. List and give an example of each of the mostly widely suspected causes of cancer.

4. List the risk factors for CVD and describe their contribution to the disease process.

5. Describe a myocardial infarction, the possible immediate causes, and what can be done to assist the heart attack victim.

6. List the seven nutritional guidelines for cancer prevention proposed by the ACS.

7. Describe the process by which malignant and benign tumors develop and how cancer spreads through the body system.

8. Describe the typical classifications of cancer and the significance of level and stage of development.

9. Describe the available cancer treatment options.

10. Describe the Type-A personality as it relates to CVD.

Fill-in-the-Blank

1. High blood pressure that cannot be attributed to any specific cause is known as _____ _____.

2. Cancerous tumors are referred to as _____ and noncancerous tumors are termed _____.

3. Cancer tumors spread to other organs by a process known as _____.

4. Heart sounds made as a result of blood pressing through irregular valve closures are called _____.

5. Mild forms of stroke are called _____ and are often indications of an impending stroke.

Multiple Choice

1. The leading cause of death in the United States is:
    a. Strokes
    b. Transient Ischemic Attacks
    c. Cardiovascular Disease
    d. Cancer

2. Physicians who specialize in the treatment of malignancies are:
    a. Oncologists
    b. Internalists
    c. Cancerologists
    d. Epidemiologists

3. The greatest alterable risk factor for CVD is:
   a. Smoking
   b. Diet
   c. Exercise
   d. Hypertension

4. The most common occupational carcinogen is:
   a. Herbicides
   b. Pesticides
   c. Coal tars
   d. Asbestos

5. The blood pressure value that refers to the pressure being applied to the walls of the arteries when the heart contracts is called:
   a. Diastolic pressure
   b. Systolic pressure
   c. Normal pressure
   d. Contraction pressure

6. Damage resulting from a blockage of the normal blood supply to the heart is:
   a. A stroke
   b. A coronary thrombosis
   c. A myocardial infarction
   d. Angina pectoris

7. Cancer of the blood-forming parts of the body, particularly the bone marrow and spleen is:
   a. Leukemia
   b. Sarcoma
   c. Malignant Melanoma
   d. Carcinomas

8. The treatment of cancer that uses drugs to kill cancerous cells is called:
   a. Immunotherapy
   b. Radiotherapy
   c. Chemotherapy
   d. None of the above

9. The diagnostic technique in which a needle-thin catheter is threaded through blocked heart arteries, a dye injected, and an X-ray of the block area is taken, is called:
   a. Angiography
   b. Angioplasty
   c. Electrocardiogram
   d. Positron Emission Tomography

10. A large group of diseases characterized by uncontrolled growth and spread of abnormal cells is called:
    a. Mutant cells
    b. Neoplasm
    c. Carcinogens
    d. Cancer

CHAPTER 14

INFECTIOUS AND NONINFECTIOUS DISEASES

CHAPTER OVERVIEW

Attention to health for Americans had much of its beginnings in initiatives to control communicable diseases through programs of research, immunization, and personal hygiene. Progress in these efforts reduced the threat of many infectious diseases and, in some cases, totally eradicated serious contagions. Concurrently, substantial attention shifted to noninfectious health threats; however, the changing nature of infectious pathogens has placed new and critical demands on programs of disease prevention and control. Likewise, a myriad of chronic maladies hold the potential for a disruptive and debilitating impact on our quality of life. These conditions usually develop over a long period of time and are not transmitted by any pathogen or by any form of personal contact. Understanding the major common characteristics of these diseases can help us prevent conditions that can often cause us the most pain, suffering, and disability. Chapter 14 explores the causes, diagnosis, treatment, and prevention of communicable diseases. You are familiarized with the nature of pathogens, the body's immune system, sexually transmitted diseases (STDs), and other common communicable diseases. Of particular interest is a discussion of acquired immune deficiency syndrome (AIDS). Furthermore, Chapter 14 discusses the role of lifestyle and personal health habits that contribute to the increased incidence of chronic diseases and the preventive measures that can be taken to ensure a high quality of living.

LEARNING OBJECTIVES

Upon completion of Chapter 14 you should be able to:

1. Explain the roles of agent, host, and environment in the disease process.
2. List, describe, and give examples of risk factors that contribute to the disease process.
3. List and describe the categories of human pathogens, their mode of transmission, examples of causative microorganisms and associated diseases, and approaches to prevention and treatment.
4. Discuss the role of the immune system in the body's defensive response to disease.
5. Describe the following STDs in terms of causative pathogen, symptoms and signs, disease process, complications, diagnosis, treatment, and prevention: chlamydia gonorrhea, syphilis, pubic lice, venereal warts, candidiasis, trichomoniasis, UTIs, and genital herpes.
6. Discuss AIDS in terms of the scope of the problem, causative pathogen, disease process, symptoms and signs, complications, at-risk groups, modes of transmission, treatment, and prevention.

7. Describe the following respiratory disorders in terms of cause, disease process, treatment, and prevention: allergies, hay fever, asthma, emphysema, and chronic bronchitis.
8. Differentiate between the most common forms of headaches and their treatments.
9. Discuss the possible causes and common approaches to treatment of epilepsy.
10. Describe fibrocystic disease, PMS, and endometriosis in terms of cause, symptoms and signs, and treatment.
11. Describe the following disorders in terms of cause, disease process, signs and symptoms, and treatment: diabetes, colitis, diverticulosis, peptic ulcers, and gallbladder disease.
12. Describe and differentiate between the different forms of arthritis.
13. Discuss low back pain in terms of the scope of the problem, risk factors, prevention, and treatment.
14. Describe Chronic Fatigue Syndrome in terms of its cause, symptoms and signs, and treatment.
15. Describe Sudden Infant Syndrome, its causes, and preventive measures.

KEY TERMS

Acquired Immunity
AIDS
Alveoli
Anaerobic
Antibodies
Antigens
ARC
Arthritis
Asthma
Asymptomatic
Bacteria
Botulism
Candidiasis (Monoiliasis)
Chancre
Chlamydia
Chronic Bronchitis
Chronic Fatigue Syndrome
Colitis
Condylomas
Conjunctivitis
Diabetes
Diverticulosis
Emphysema
Endometriosis
Epidermis
Epilepsy
Fungi
Genital Herpes

Iarogenic Diseases
Immunity
Incubation Period
Influenza
Insulin
Interferon
Low Back Pain (LBP)
Lymphocytes
Measles
Migraine Headaches
Natural Immunity
Pasteurization
Pathogen
Penicillin
Peptic Ulcers
Periodontal Disease
PID
Pneumonia
Premenstrual Syndrome (PMS)
Protazoa
Pubic Lice
Rabies
Rickettsia
Salmonellosis
Seroconversion
Sickle Cell Anemia
Slow Viral Infections
Staphylococci

EXPLORING YOUR ACCESS TO HEALTH

"Personal Immunization Record"

This is an exercise to check your active immunization history. From your best recollection, record the following information. Perhaps consult with your parents or physicians who may have records of your immunizations and childhood diseases.

Immunization	Date	Booster?
Smallpox		
Rubella		
Mumps		
Measles		
Polio		
Tetanus		
Pertussis		
Diphtheria		

Childhood Diseases or Immunizations	Date	Notes
Influenza		
TB		
Typhoid		
Cholera		
Hepatitis		
Strep		

Measles

Chickenpox

Scoring: Please turn to the exercise entitled "Personal Immunity."

ASSESSING HEALTH

1. **Communicable Disease Matrix**. Develop a matrix of the communicable diseases discussed in your textbook. For each disease, indicate the pathogen, mode of transmission, symptoms and signs, treatment, and preventive measures. Make a copy of this page for additional entries.

2. **SID Matrix**. Construct another matrix, listing the sexually transmitted diseases discussed in your textbook. Indicate their causative pathogens, symptoms and signs, complications, treatment, and prevention. Make a copy of this page for additional entries.

3. **Personal Immunity**. Review your entries on the "Personal Immunization Record." You may also want to check any instances of passive acquired immunity. Read the section on immunity in your textbook to better understand your immunization history and the differences between natural, active acquired, and passive immunity.

4. **Looking Further**. Investigate the programs and services in your community that are directed at sexually transmitted diseases.

   a. What resources are available for diagnosis and treatment of STDs?

   b. What resources are available to assist persons suffering from AIDS, ARC, or those tested as HIV positive?

   c. Visit your local American Red Cross Blood Center and ask about procedures used to screen for AIDs. If you have no personal objections, volunteer to donate blood. It is an easy way to be tested for AIDS antibodies, and blood donation is a vital service to the community. Remember that giving blood does not place one at risk of contracting AIDS.

   d. Prepare a list of questions about AIDS and call one or more of the following telephone "hotline" information services. They will be happy to answer your questions in a candid and sensitive manner.

   Centers for Disease Control Hotline: 1-800-342-AIDS U.S. Public Health Service Hotline: 1-800-447-AIDS National Gay Task Force and AIDS Crisis Hotline: 1-800-221-7044

REVIEW TEST

Short Answer

1. Briefly describe grand mal, petit mal, psychomotor, and Jacksonian seizures.

2. Briefly describe the most plausible cause of PMS and the arguments that support and refute this contention.

3. Briefly discuss the contribution of lifestyle to the development infectious disease.

4. Briefly explain how fever acts as a form of protection in systemic infections.

5. List the seven factors that health experts believe contribute to low back pain.

6. Describe and differentiate between the different forms of arthritis.

7. List seven generally accepted recommendations for reducing personal risks for AIDS.

8. Discuss the role of the immune system in the body's defensive response to disease.

9. Describe the roles of agent, host, and environment in the disease process.

10. Compare and contrast allergies, hay fever, and asthma, in terms of their cause, disease process, treatment, and prevention.

Fill-in-the-Blank

1. _____ theory demonstrated the relationship between pathogenic microorganisms and disease development.

2. _____ are chemical substances that dilate blood vessels, increase mucus secretions, cause tissues to swell and produce other allergylike symptoms.

3. ._____ and _____ are the forms of Lymphocyte involved in the immune response.

4. _____ is the general term for a family of viral diseases characterized by sores or eruptions on the skin.

5. _____ is a respiratory disorder in which the airway becomes so inflamed and swollen that normal respiratory function is impaired.

Multiple Choice

1. The process that heats fluids such as milk to a temperature just below the boiling point to destroy bacteria is called:
   a. Sterilization
   b. Pasteurization
   c. Disinfection
   d. Listerization

2. Organisms that normally live within the human host are called:
   a. Pathogens
   b. Exogenous microorganisms
   c. Endogenous microorganisms
   d. Infectious microorganisms

3. A respiratory disease in which the alveoli become distended or ruptured and are no longer functional is known as:
   a. Asthma
   b. Hay fever
   c. Emphysema
   d. Chronic Bronchitis

4. Staphylococcal infection is a form of:
   a. Rickettsia infections
   b. Fungi infections
   c. Viral infections
   d. Bacterial infections

5. Epilepsy is:
   a. Localized headaches on only one side of the head
   b. A neurological disorder caused by abnormal electrical brain activity
   c. Characterized by excruciating pain that lasts for minutes or hours
   d. A hereditary disease that is more common in women than men

6. Symptoms for diabetes include all of the following except:
   a. Excessive thirst
   b. Hypoglycemia
   c. Frequent urination
   d. Skin eruptions

7. When the gallbladder has been repeatedly irritated and reduces its ability to release bile, a disease that can result is:
   a. Diverticulosis
   b. Colitis
   c. Cholecystitis
   d. Appendicitis

8. White blood cells that aid in the antigen-antibody response are known as:
   a. Antigens
   b. Lymphocytes
   c. Phagocytes
   d. Erythrocytes

9. The most common sexually transmitted disease (STD) is:
   a. Chlamydia
   b. Nongonococcal urethritis (NGU)
   c. Syphilis
   d. Genital herpes

10. The leading cause of death among infants one week to one year of age is:
    a. Pneumonia
    b. Congenital heart disorders
    c. Sudden infant death syndrome
    d. Child abuse

CHAPTER 15

SUCCESSFUL LIFE TRANSITIONS

CHAPTER OVERVIEW

As we grow older, we experience many physical and psychological transitions that are a part of the aging process. The changing age structure of society poses challenges to develop practices and policies that will focus upon healthful and productive aging. Chapter 15 explores the relationship between aging and health with emphasis on the physical, mental, emotional, and social dimensions of the aging process. As our population continues to age, a host of problems and afflictions may arise for some elderly. Chapter 15 describes the "typical" aging changes that we can reasonably expect to happen to ourselves as we continue to grow older. Furthermore, we can optimize our physical and psychological health by taking responsible actions to promote optimal physical, mental, and social well-being. Chapter 15 also examines our final transition, that of death and dying. The definitions of death are discussed and how these definitions have been modified to be consistent with innovations in medical life-support technology and life itself. Chapter 15 explores the stages of dying as described by Elisabeth Kubler-Ross. This chapter describes the normal grief reactions and when it is appropriate to seek counseling for unresolved grief. Chapter 15 concludes with special ethical concerns of the right to die, including rational suicide, dyathanasia, and euthanasia.

LEARNING OBJECTIVES

Upon completion of Chapter 15 you should be able to:

1. Discuss the stud of aging and the categories for spedific age-related haracteristics.
2. Discuss today's elderly population in terms of age, size, social and health care costs, housing and living arrangements, abuse and ethical and moral considerations.
3. Discuss the special problems associated with alcohol and drug use, self-medicating, vitamin and mineral supplementing, and mental health.
4. Describe the aging process in terms of physiology, sexuality, and cognition, and the contribution of environment versus biology.
5. Discuss the problem of osteoporosis, its prevention, treatment, and the associated controversies.
6. List and describe the factors which should be attended to for successful aging.
7. Differentiate between death and dying.
8. Describe biological, apparent, functional, local, somatic, and brain death.
9. Discuss the use of a "flat" EEG in determining death and the death determination rules for organ donor transplants.
10. List and describe the five stages of dying suggested by Kubler-Ross.

11. List the guidelines for communicating with the dying and their families.
12. Describe the functions of bereavement, grief, and mourning in coping with loss.
13. Explain the purpose of hospice and describe its eight characteristics.
14. Differentiate between living, holographic, and legally written wills.
15. Explain what is meant by rational suicide, dyathanasia, and euthanasia and discuss the ethical concerns regarding the right to die.

KEY TERMS

Ageism	Gerontology
Aging	Glaucoma
Alzheimer's Disease	Grief
Autoimmune Theory	Grief Work
Bereavement	Hospice
Cataracts	Intestate
Death	Mourning
Dyathanasia	Osteoporosis
Dying	Rigor Mortis
Dying Trajectory	Senility
Electroencephalogram	Social Security
Euthanasia	Thanatology

EXPLORING YOUR A ACCESS TO HEALTH

"How Long Will You Live?"

Complete this assessment by beginning with the number 72 and subtracting and adding the numbers indicated in the items that apply to you.

Personal Facts

                                                                                                                  72

1. If you are male, subtract 3.
2. If female, add 4.
3. If you live in an urban area with a population over 2 million, subtract 2.
4. If you live in a town under 10,000 or on a farm, add 2.
5. If any grandparent lived to 85, add 2.
6. If all four grandparents lived to 80, add 6.
7. If either parent died of a stroke or heart attack before the age of 50, subtract 4.
8. If any parent, brother, or sister under 50 has (or had) cancer or a heart condition, or has had diabetes since childhood, subtract 3.
9. Do you earn over $50,000 a year? Subtract 2.

10. If you finished college, add 1. If you have a graduate or professional degree, add 2 more. _____
11. If you are 65 or older and still working, add 3. _____
12. If you live with a spouse or friend, add 5. If not, subtract 1 for every ten years alone since 25. _____

Lifestyle Status

13. If you work behind desk, subtract 3.
14. If your work requires regular, heavy physical labor, add 3. _____
15. If you exercise strenuously (tennis, running, swimming etc.) five times a week for at least a half-hour, add 4. Two or three times a week, add 2. _____
16. Do you sleep more than ten hours each night? Subtract 4. _____
17. Are you intense, aggressive, easily angered? Subtract 3. _____
18. Are you easy going and relaxed? Add 3. _____
19. Are you happy? Add 1. Unhappy? Subtract 2. _____
20. Have you had a speeding ticket in the past year? Subtract 1. _____
21. Do you smoke more than two packs a day? Subtract 8. One to two packs? Subtract 6. One-half to one? Subtract 3. _____
22. Do you drink the equivalent of 1 1/2 oz. of liquor a day? Subtract 1. _____
23. Are you overweight by 50 lbs. or more? Subtract 8. By 30 to 50 lbs? Subtract 4. By 10 to 30 lbs? Subtract 2. _____
24. If you are a man over 40 and have annual checkups, add 2. _____
25. If you are a woman and see a gynecologist once a year, add 2. _____

Age Adjustment

26. If you are between 30 and 40, add 2. _____
27. If you are between 40 and 50, add 3. _____
28. If you are between 50 and 70, add 4. _____
29. If you are over 70, add 5. _____

Scoring

Total your score to get you life expectancy. Go to the exercise entitled "Life Expectancy" for your interpretation and application of your score.

Source: Allen, R.F., & Linde, S. (1981). *Life Again: The Exciting New Program That Will Change Your Health and Your Life.* New York: Appleton-Century-Crofts. Used with permission of Prentice Hall, Inc.

"You and Death Questionnaire"

Carefully consider each question and assess your attitudes toward death by circling the letter of the answer that best reflects how you feel.

1. Who died in your first personal involvement with death?
   a. Grandparent or great-grandparent
   b. Parent
   c. Brother or sister
   d. Other family member
   e. Friend or acquaintance
   f. Stranger
   g. Public figure
   h. Animal

2. To the best of your memory, at what age were you first aware of death?
   a. Under 3
   b. 3 to 5
   c. 5 to 10
   d. 10 or older

3. When you were a child, how was death talked about in your family?
   a. Openly
   b. With some sense of discomfort
   c. Only when necessary and then with an attempt to exclude the children.
   d. As though it were a taboo subject
   e. Never recall any discussion

4. Which of the following best describes your childhood conception of death?
   a. Heaven-and-hell concept
   b. After-life
   c. Death as a sleep
   d. Cessation of all physical and mental activity
   e. Mysterious and unknowable
   f. Something other than the above
   g. No conception
   h. Can't remember

5. To what extent do you believe in a life after death?
   a. Strongly believe in it
   b. Tend to believe it
   c. Uncertain
   d. Tend to doubt it
   e. Convinced it does not exist

6. Regardless of your belief about life after death, what is your wish about it?
   a. I strongly wish there were a life after death
   b. I am indifferent as to whether there is a life after death
   c. I definitely prefer that there not be a life after death

7. Has there been a time in your life when you wanted to die?
    a. Yes, mainly because of great at physical pain
    b. Yes, mainly because of great emotional upset
    c. Yes, mainly to escape an intolerable social or interpersonal situation
    d. Yes, mainly because of great embarrassment
    e. Yes, for a reason other than above
    f. No

8. What does death mean to you?
    a. The end; the final process of life
    b. The beginning of life after death; a transition, a new beginning
    c. A joining of the spirit with a universal cosmic consciousness
    d. A kind of endless sleep; rest and peace
    e. Termination of this life but with survival of the spirit
    f. Don't know
    g. Other (specify) _____

9. What aspect of your death is the most distasteful to you?
    a. I could no longer have any experiences
    b. I am afraid of what might happen to my body after death
    c. I am uncertain as to what might happen to me if there is a life after death
    d. I could no longer provide for my dependents
    e. It would cause grief to my relatives and friends
    f. All my plans and projects would come to an end
    g. The process of dying might be painful
    h. Other (specify) _____

10. How do you rate your present physical health?
    a. Excellent
    b. Very good
    c. Moderately good
    d. Moderately poor
    e. Extremely poor

11. How do you rate your present mental health?
    a. Excellent
    b. Very good
    c. Moderately good
    d. Moderately poor
    e. Extremely poor

12. Based on your present feelings, what is the probability of your taking your own life in the near future?
    a. Extremely high (I feel very much like killing myself)
    b. Moderately high
    c. Between high and low
    d. Moderately low
    e. Extremely low (very improbable that I would kill myself)

13. In your opinion, at what age are people most afraid of death?
    a. Up to 12 years
    b. 13 to 19 year
    c. 20 to 29 years
    d. 30 to 39 years
    e. 40 to 49 years
    f. 50 to 59 years
    g. 60 to 69 years
    h. 70 years and over

14. When you think of your own death (or when circumstances make you realize your own mortality), how do you feel?
    a. Fearful
    b. Discouraged
    c. Depressed
    d. Purposeless
    e. Resolved, in relation to life
    f. Pleasure, in being alive
    g. Other (specify) _____

15. What is your present orientation to your own death?
    a. Death-seeker
    b. Discouraged
    c. Depressed
    d. Purposeless
    e. Resolved, in relation to life
    f. Death-fearer

16. If you were told you had a terminal disease and a limited time to live, how would you want to spend your time until you died?
    a. I would make a marked change in my lifestyle; satisfy hedonistic needs (travel, sex, drugs, other experiences).
    b. I would become more withdrawn; reading, contemplating or praying.
    c. I would shift from my own needs to a concern for others (family, friends).
    d. I would attempt to complete projects; tie up loose ends.
    e. I would make little or no change in my lifestyle.
    f. I would try to do one very important thing.
    g. I might consider committing suicide.
    h. I would do none of these.

17. How do you feel about having an autopsy done on your body?
    a. Approve
    b. Don't care one way or the other
    c. Disapprove
    d. Strongly disapprove

Scoring

Proceed to the exercise entitled, "Attitudes Toward Death."

Source: Schneidman, E. (August, 1970). You and death questionnaire. *Psychology Today.* Reprinted by permission.

ASSESSING HEALTH

1. **Preparing for Aging.** Aging is an inevitable process of life. Consideration of the consequent physical and social changes gives rise to expectations for our personal aging and that of loved ones. After completing the "Are You Preparing for Old Age" questionnaire in your textbook, give some thought to why you completed each statement in that way. Are your expectations for aging bright or dismal? Why?

2. **Life Expectancy.** The health and longevity of grandparents, parents, and siblings and your own lifestyle can have predictive value in forecasting your life expectancy. The "How Long Will You Live?" assessment accounts for these factors in giving you an estimate of the age to which you can expect to live. However, the sum of your calculations is not written in stone. The real value of this assessment is that given your heredity, any other loss of points clearly reveals changes you can make to add points and therefore years to your predicted life expectancy. Review the items for which you lost points and summarize the changes you can make to increase the estimate of your longevity.

3. **Attitudes Toward Death.** Examine your responses to the "You And Death Questionnaire." If your answers tend to reflect uncomfortable feelings about death, consider why you feel this way. How could you change your attitudes to relieve your discomfort? Perhaps, discuss your feelings with classmates, friends, and/or family.

4. **Funeral Planning.** Visit a funeral home in your home community and investigate possible arrangements as if you were planning your own funeral. Consider the various options available in terms of cost, services provided, and payment alternatives.

REVIEW TEST

Short Answer

1. Explain what is meant by the term "flat" EEG in determining death and the death determination rules for organ donor transplants.

2. Briefly describe the physiological changes in eyesight, the heart and lungs, hearing, and taste associated with aging.

3. Briefly discuss the controversies produced by recent research on osteoporosis.

4. List three sexual changes which generally occur with aging for males and females.

5. Briefly describe what changes in intelligence and memory we can expect with aging.

6. Describe the five stages of dying suggested by Kubler-Ross.

7. Describe the functions of bereavement, grief, and mourning in coping with loss.

8. Compare and contrast the terms "old" and "aging."

9. Explain the purpose of hospice and list its eight characteristics.

10. Differentiate between living, holographic, and legally written wills.

Fill-in-the-Blank

1. A handwritten and unwitnessed will is called a(n) _____ will.

2. _____ is the study of individual and collective aging process.

3. A permanent cessation of all vital functions is called _____.

4. _____ is the study of death and dying.

5. Some research indicates that _____ may be the leading mental health problem for the elderly.

Multiple Choice

1. Rigor mortis is associated with:
   a. Local death
   b. Cell death
   c. Biological death
   d. Brain death

2. The relative age or condition of a person's organs and body systems is:
   a. Functional age
   b. Psychological age
   c. Legal age
   d. Biological age

3. A federal system of insurance for elderly persons financed by employees, employers, and the government is known as:
   a. Federal Insurance Compensation
   b. Social Security
   c. National Comprehensive Medical Insurance
   d. Federal Disability Insurance

4. An electroencephalogram is used to determine:
   a. Local death
   b. Cell death
   c. Biological death
   d. Brain death

5. A mental state of distress that occurs in reaction to the loss of a loved one is called:
   a. Bereavement
   b. Mourning
   c. Grief
   d. Denial

6. Alzheimer's Disease is characterized by:
   a. Forgetfulness, memory loss, disorientation
   b. Agitation and restlessness
   c. Loss of control of bodily functions
   d. All of the above

7. As a normal consequence of aging:
   a. The sense of taste increases so that less spices are needed to enhance food flavor
   b. Resting heart rate increases
   c. Nose grows wider and longer
   d. The ability to hear high frequency sounds improves

8. A common grief reaction is:
   a. A feeling of tightness in the throat
   b. Choking and shortness of breath
   c. Disrupted sleeping patterns
   d. All of the above

9. In order to enhance the aging process, it is important to:
   a. Exercise regularly
   b. Control alcohol consumption
   c. Maintain an appropriate diet
   d. All of the above

10. The disposition of human remains by burial without formal viewing, visitation, or ceremony with the body present, except for a graveside service is called:
    a. Direct cremation
    b. Immediate burial
    c. Direct burial
    d. Direct internment

CHAPTER 16

ENVIRONMENTAL HEALTH

CHAPTER OVERVIEW

Personal efforts to promote well-being are too often limited to factors of lifestyle while overlooking the significant impact of environmental forces and personal actions that can be taken to maximize healthy surroundings. Manage-ment of our environment and its resources is a priority as the century draws to a close. While the magnitude of environmental problems globally is over-whelming, individuals must begin to behave in environmentally responsible ways to protect the earth's resources. Chapter 16 explores the problems, challenges, and solutions related to environmental health. The discussion focuses upon environmental issues related to population: air, water, waste, radiation, and nuclear pollution. Finally, Chapter 16 outlines specific actions we can take to preserve our personal and larger environments.

LEARNING OBJECTIVES

Upon completion of Chapter 16 you should be able to:

1. Describe the significance of population growth in environmental problems and approaches to population stabilization.
2. Describe the effects of air pollution on plant, animal, and human life.
3. Explain the function of the EPA in monitoring air quality standards.
4. List the various types of air pollution and describe their effects on the environment and health.
5. List and describe examples of water pollution and the effects on the environment and health.
6. Describe the effects of noise pollution.
7. Describe the hazardous waste disposal problem and its solutions.
8. Describe problems associated with sewage and solid waste disposal and corresponding remedies.
9. Describe the health risks posed by radiation and nuclear pollution, potential sources of such pollution, and examples which illustrate these threats.
10. Describe four ways that individuals can take action to positively impact the environment.

KEY TERMS

Acid Deposition
Carbon Monoxide
Chlorofluorocarbons
Deep-Well Injection
Dioxin
Fission
Greenhouse Gases
Half-Life

Nuclear Winter
Ozone
Particulates
Polychlorinated Biphenyls (PCBs)
Pesticides
Photochemical Smog
Radiation
Rads

Hydrocarbons
Incineration
Leachate
Lead
Nitrogen Dioxide

Solid Waste
Secure Landfills
Sulfur Dioxide
Temperature Inversion

EXPLORING YOUR ACCESS TO HEALTH

"Environmental Sensitivity Assessment"

Respond to each question by indicating "YES" or "NO."

1. Do you smoke? _____
2. Do you litter? _____
3. Do you waste electricity? _____
4. Do you use phosphate detergents? _____
5. Do you plan on having more than two children? _____
6. Do you like to play music as loud as possible? _____
7. Do you only buy blemish-free farm produce? _____
8. Do you use spray cans? _____
9. Do you use throw-away aluminum cans instead of returnable bottles? _____
10. Do you burn leaves or trash? _____
11. Do you idle your automobile needlessly? _____
12. Do you use colored tissues, colored paper, or colored napkins? _____
13. Do you waste water via lengthy showers, dishwashing, or watering of lawns? _____
14. Do you purchase liquids sold in opaque white plastic containers? _____
15. Do you use paper products instead of cloth handkerchiefs, napkins, and towels? _____

Scoring

Note the questions to which you answered "YES" and proceed to the "Environmental Sensitivity" exercise.

Source: Kammerman, S., Doyle, K., Valois, R., & Cox, S. (1983). *Wellness R.S.V.P.* (2nd ed.). Menlo Park: Benjamin/Cummings, 142 & 143. Reprinted by permission.

ASSESSING HEALTH

1. **Environmental Sensitivity**. Review your responses to the "Environmental Sensitivity Assessment." If you responded "YES" to any of these questions, consider how you could change your behaviors to help protect the environment. Comments on each question are provided below so you may better understand your personal contribution to environmental pollution.

    1. The inhalation of smoke increases your risk for lung diseases; smoke also pollutes the air, thereby affecting persons around you.

    2. Litter may be classified as either solid waste or visual blight. Only through individual effort can this form of pollution be managed.

    3. Electrical power consumption affects the thermal water pollution loads at electrical generating plants. One simple way to lower your electricity consumption is to switch light bulbs not used for reading to lower wattage bulbs.

    4. A great deal of pollution comes from detergent phosphates. The new biodegradable detergents merely cut down the foam, i.e., they still contain phosphates, which fertilize algae and, in turn, reduce the supply of oxygen necessary to support other forms of life in streams, lakes, and oceans.

    5. With the population size growing daily, if you want to have more than two children in your family, you should consider adopting the rest.

    6. Learn to enjoy music at lower volumes. Noise pollution over a period of time will lead to irreversible hearing losses.

    7. Accept produce with blemishes caused by insects or minor plant diseases. This will reduce the number of farmers who are forced to use pesticides that merely save the appearance of the produce.

    8. Fluorocarbon propellants are depleting the ozone layer and are also increasing the future incidence of skin cancer. Ozone absorbs solar ultraviolet rays and without it variations in weather, food supply, and disease will be inevitable.

    9. If aluminum cans are recycled in your community, all is well. But if they are discarded, use returnable bottles, and make efforts to organize a community recycling program.

    10. Rather than burning leaves, start your own compost pile to return the nutrients in leaves to the soil. Trash is solid waste and should be handled through sanitary landfill.

    11. The automobile is the single greatest source of air pollution. If you will be waiting more than one minute, shut your automobile off.

    12. By buying these colored paper products, you are basically supporting the release of dyes into lakes and streams, polluting waters visually and biologically. Try to reduce or eliminate such purchases.

    13. North America has the best fresh water supply in the world but remember that if you waste this invaluable resource, future generations may be forced to restrict personal consumption. To conserve water, think about taking

shorter showers, using drought-resistant landscaping, conserving rinse water during dishwashing, and reducing the amount of water used in toilets by placing several bricks in each flush tank.

14. Do not purchase liquids sold in opaque white plastic containers. This is polyvinyl chloride. It is a hazardous substance; when burned it can destroy nearby vegetation, the insides of incinerators, and the lining of your lungs if inhaled.

15. Paper comes from wood, so using paper excessively threatens the existence of our national forests. Take the time and use handkerchiefs, cloth napkins, and towels.

Source: Kammerman, S., et. al. (1983). *Wellness R.S.V.P.* (2nd ed.). Menlo Park: Benjamin/Cummings, 142 & 143. Reprinted by permission.

2. **Resources for Environmental Action.** Write the agencies listed in your textbook and request information on environmental health and their activities to promote environmental protection.

REVIEW TEST

Short Answer

1. Briefly describe the problems associated with zero population growth.

2. List three approaches to fighting air pollution.

3. Describe the effects of air pollution on plant, animal, and human life.

4. List the various types of air pollution and describe their effects on the environment and health.

5. Briefly discuss what must be done to solve the hazardous waste disposal problem.

6. List what individuals can do to help manage solid waste disposal.

7. Differentiate between sound and noise.

8. Describe the effects of noise pollution.

9. Briefly describe the problems associated with sewage and solid waste and steps to be taken to remedy these problems.

10. Briefly describe the theoretical situation of a nuclear winter and the likely impact on the environment.

Fill-in-the-Blank

1. _____ _____ are chemical compounds that contain carbon and hydrogen.

2. Combustion of fuels containing sulfur are the most common sources of sulfur _____ pollutants.

3. _____ matter is the term used to describe nongaseous air pollutants.

4. Although once called a "miracle fiber," _____ is now known to contribute to serious lung disease.

5. A substance is said to be _____ when it emits high-energy particles from the nuclei of its atoms.

Multiple Choice

1. Ozone is:
    a. Formed when nitrogen dioxide reacts with hydrogen chloride
    b. Is found in motor vehicle exhaust
    c. A brown, hazy mix of particulates and gases
    d. A by-product of coal-powered electrical generated stations

2. The primary origin of carbon monoxide is:
    a. Coal -powered electrical generated stations
    b. Electrical utility boilers
    c. Dry cleaners
    d. Motor vehicle emissions

3. Precipitation that has fallen through acidic air pollutants, particularly those containing sulfur dioxides and nitrogen dioxides is known as:
    a. Ozone
    b. Acid deposition
    c. Photochemical smog
    d. Temperature inversion

4. Nongaseous air pollutants that are tiny solid particles or liquid droplets which are suspended in the air are called:
    a. Asbestos
    b. Particulates
    c. Radon
    d. Formaldehyde

5. Chlorofluorocarbons, chemicals that contribute to the depletion of the ozone, are found in:
    a. Hair spray
    b. Deodorants
    c. Styrofoam
    d. All of the above

6. Industrial chemicals used in electrical transformers, lubricants, and plastics that can cause cancer are known as:
    a. Dioxins
    b. Polychlorinated biphenyls (PCBs)
    c. Pesticides
    d. Trichlorethylene (TCE)

7. A symptom of noise-related distress is:
    a. Decreased blood pressure
    b. Increased productivity
    c. Decreased cholesterol levels
    d. Increased secretion of adrenaline

8. A principal method for disposal of hazardous waste is(are):
   a. Secure landfill
   b. Incineration
   c. Deep-well injection
   d. All of the above

9. The recommended maximum "safe" dosage of radiation is:
   a. 0.5 rads to 5 rads per year
   b. 25 rads to 35 rads per year
   c. 50 rads to 60 rads per year
   d. 100 rads to 200 rads per year

10. The splitting of atoms that results in the release of atomic energy is called:
    a. Radiation
    b. Radiation absorbed doses
    c. Fission
    d. Cosmic rays

APPENDIX

FIRST AID AND EMERGENCY CARE

CHAPTER OVERVIEW

Emergencies can occur at any time and in any place. Being prepared for situations and being able to administer immediate basic care can save lives. Its important to know when to call for help and what information to give EMS personnel that can save someone's life. The Appendix describes the EMS system and the information that is invaluable for alerting emergency personnel about the situation. The Appendix further describes the procedures for such common life threatening situations as cardiovascular and respiratory emergencies, choking, bleeding, burns, shock, poisoning, sprains, fractures, head injuries, and heat and cold injuries. Finally, the Appendix provides a list of the basic supplies needed for a first aid kit.

LEARNING OBJECTIVES

Upon completion of the Appendix you should be able to:

1. Describe the local Emergency Medical System and the questions you should be prepared to answer when accessing the system.
2. Discuss liability and the "Good Samaritan" laws.
3. Describe CPR and rescue breathing procedures.
4. Briefly describe the Heimlich method for assisting a choking victim, both conscious and unconscious.
5. Discuss three major procedures to control external bleeding.
6. Describe the symptoms and how treat the following emergency situations: burns, shock, poisoning, sprains, fractures, head injuries, frostbite, hypothermia, heat stroke, and heat exhaustion.
7. Describe the supplies that should be included in a basic first aid kit.

KEY TERMS

Cardiopulmonary Resuscitation	Heat Exhaustion
Good Samaritan Laws	Heat Stroke
Fractures	Hypothermia
Frostbite	Shock
Head Injury	Sprains
Heat Cramps	

EXPLORING YOUR ACCESS TO HEALTH

"Are You Prepared?"

Emergencies can occur at any time and at any place. Would you be able to respond to the following situations?

	Yes	No

1. While at a restaurant, you notice a man holding his throat and is unable to breath or talk. He is choking on his food. _____ _____

2. While driving home one evening you come upon an auto accident that has just occurred. Several people are injured and help has not arrived yet. _____ _____

3. Your neighbor has cut his leg badly with a skill saw and is bleeding badly. _____ _____

4. While at the grocery store, you are standing next to a man who begins complaining that he is having chest pains. _____ _____

If you responded No to any of the above questions, proceed to the Emergency Preparedness in the following section.

ASSESSING HEALTH

1. **Emergency Preparedness.** Based on the list of first aid supplies in your textbook, construct a basic first aid kit. Do you have all of the supplies that you would need in the event of an emergency?

2. **Looking Further.** Enroll in a CPR and first aid course through one of your local agencies, such as the American Red Cross, American Heart Association, Paramed Foundation, or other organization for information on CPR and first aid courses.

REVIEW TEST

Short Answer

1. Briefly list the questions that you should be ready to answer when calling for emergency assistance.

2. Discuss the "Good Samaritan" laws for liability in administering first aid.

3. List the steps that should be followed in performing mouth-to-mouth resuscitation..

4. Briefly describe cardiopulmonary resuscitation.

5. Briefly describe the three major ways to control external bleeding.

6. List the symptoms of shock.

7. Briefly discuss the steps to follow in rendering first aid for electrical shock.

8. List the contents of a basic first aid kit.

9. Briefly describe the three common heat-related emergencies

10. Describe frostbite and list the steps to be followed for it's treatment.

Fill-in-the-Blank

1. If someone has stopped breathing, you should perform _____.

2. The _____ _____ is used for choking victims.

3. _____ _____ are places over a bone where arteries are close to the skin.

4. ____% of poisonings occur in children under age 5.

5. When ligaments and other tissues around a joint are stretched or torn, _____ can result.

Multiple Choice

1. Damage to body tissues caused by intense cold are called:
    a. Hypothermia
    b. Frostbite
    c. Hyperthermia
    d. Cold exhaustion

2. When the victim is not breathing and does not have a pulse, it is appropriate to perform:
    a. Mouth-to-mouth resuscitation
    b. Heimlich maneuver
    c. Cardiopulmonary resuscitation
    d. Direct pressure to the radial artery

3. The universal sign for choking is:
    a. Clasping of the throat with one or both hands
    b. Not being able to talk
    c. Noisy whistles
    d. Difficulty breathing

4. Which of the following is *not* a symptom of internal bleeding:
    a. Symptoms of shock
    b. Blood in urine
    c. Increased appetite
    d. Black, tarlike stools

5. Any deformity of an injured body part usually signals:
   a. Internal bleeding
   b. Sprains
   c. Shock
   d. Fractures

6. The key symptoms of hypothermia include all of the following except:
   a. Shivering
   b. Rapid breathing and heart rate
   c. Vague, slow, slurred speech
   d. Numbness and loss of feeling in extremities

7. The most serious heat-related disorder is:
   a. Hyperthermia
   b. Heat Exhaustion
   c. Heat stroke
   d. Heat cramps

8. Which of the following is not a procedure for controlling bleeding?
   a. Direct pressure
   b. Elevation
   c. Sitting the victim in a comfortable position
   d. Pressure points

9. The symptoms for shock include all of the following except:
   a. Constricted pupils
   b. Cool, moist skin
   c. Vomiting
   d. Weak, rapid pulse

10. Heat exhaustion is characterized by:
    a. Gradual fatigue and weakness
    b. Anxiety
    c. Nausea
    d. All of the above

ANSWER KEY

Chapter 1:
Fill-in-the-Blanks: (1) Health promotion (2) Quantity, Quality (3) 58% (4) Health Locus of Control (5) Readiness, Self-Efficacy, Knowledge, Motivation
Multiple Choice: (1) b (2) b (3) c (4) d (5) c (6) d (7) d (8) d (9) b (10) a

Chapter 2:
Fill-in-the-Blanks: (1) Normal (2) Continuous (3) Psychology (4) Sadness, Fear, Anger, Joy (5) Posttraumatic Stress Disorder
Multiple Choice: (1) c (2) d (3) a (4) b (5) a (6) d (7) b (8) a (9) c (10) d

Chapter 3:
Fill-in-the-Blanks: (1) Stress (2) Sympathetic, Parasympathetic (3) Control, Committment, Challenge (4) Retirement (5) Meditation
Multiple Choice: (1) b (2) c (3) a (4) c (5) b (6) d (7) a (8) c (9) a (10) b

Chapter 4:
Fill-in-the-Blanks: (1) One person takes the risk to share personal feelings, thoughts, and experiences with another (2) Trust, self-disclosure, negotiation, compromise (3) Shared financial plans, property, raising children (4) Ovaries (5) Pedophilia, Incest
Multiple Choice: (1) b (2) b (3) a (4) d (5) b (6) d (7) b (8) c (9) c (10) c

Chapter 5:
Fill-in-the-Blanks: (1) First (2) Down's Syndrome (3) Ultrasound (4) Reversible, Permanent (5) Low sperm count
Multiple Choice: 1) c (2) c (3) a (4) c (5) a (6) d (7) c (8) b (9) d (10) b

Chapter 6:
Fill-in-the-Blanks: (1) Senses (2) Essential Amino Acids (3) Fat Soluble, Water Soluble (4) Vitamin C (5) Minerals
Multiple Choice: 1) c (2) a (3) d (4) c (5) b (6) d (7) a (8) c (9) c (10) b

Chapter 7:
Fill-in-the-Blanks: (1) Hydrostatic weighing (2) Anorexia Nervosa (3) Basal metabolic rate (4) 3,500 (5) Nutrition/exercise training
Multiple Choice: 1) d (2) b (3) c (4) a (5) b (6) c (7) a (8) d (9) b (10) b

Chapter 8:
Fill-in-the-Blanks: (1) Blood glucose (2) Lactate threshold (3) Detraining (4) Catecholamines (5) Dehydration
Multiple Choice: 1) c (2) c (3) c (4) a (5) a (6) d (7) d (8) b (9) d (10) a

Chapter 9:
Fill-in-the-Blanks: (1) Concentric (2) Repetition (3) Spot reducing (4) Fat (5) Static, Isometric
Multiple Choice: 1) c (2) a (3) c (4) a (5) b (6) c (7) c (8) c (9) c (10) a

Chapter 10:
Fill-in-the-Blanks: (1) Addictive behaviors (2) Positive mood change (3) Involvement, Loss of control, Denial, Relapse (4) Nicotine (5) Denial
Multiple Choice: 1) b (2) a (3) d (4) c (5) a (6) c (7) b (8) a (9) d (10) c

Chapter 11:
Fill-in-the-Blanks: (1) Fermentation (2) Liver (3) Fetal Alcohol Syndrome (4) Carbon Monoxide (5) Tar
Multiple Choice: 1) c (2) a (3) b (4) b (5) c (6) c (7) a (8) a (9) c (10) a

Chapter 12:
   Fill-in-the-Blanks: (1) Caffeinism (2) Intolerance (3) Crack (4) Mushrooms (5) Diuretics
   Multiple Choice: 1) d (2) b (3) c (4) b (5) a (6) a (7) c (8) d (9) c (10) d

Chapter 13:
   Fill-in-the-Blanks: (1) Essential hypertension (2) Malignant, Benign (3) Metastasis (4) Murmurs (5) Transient Ischemic Attacks (TIAs)
   Multiple Choice: 1) c (2) a (3) a (4) d (5) b (6) c (7) a (8) c (9) a (10) d

Chapter 14:
   Fill-in-the-Blanks: (1) Germ (2) Histamines (3) T-Lymphocytes, B-Lymphocytes (4) Chickenpox (5) Chronic Bronchitis
   Multiple Choice: 1) b (2) c (3) c (4) d (5) b (6) b (7) c (8) b (9) a (10) c

Chapter 15:
   Fill-in-the-Blanks: (1) Holographic (2) Gerontology (3) Death (4) Thanatology (5) Depression
   Multiple Choice: 1) b (2) d (3) b (4) d (5) c (6) d (7) b (8) d (9) d (10) b

Chapter 16:
   Fill-in-the-Blanks: (1) Hydrocarbons (2) Dioxide (3) Particulates (4) Asbestos (5) Radioactive
   Multiple Choice: 1) a (2) d (3) b (4) a (5) d (6) b (7) d (8) d (9) a (10) c

Appendix:
   Fill-in-the-Blanks: (1) Mouth-to-mouth resuscitation (2) Heimlich maneuver (3) Pressure points (4) 75% (5) Sprains
   Multiple Choice: 1) b (2) c (3) a (4) c (5) d (6) b (7) c (8) c (9) a (10) d